HOW TO TONE AND TRIM YOUR TROUBLE SPOTS

NO-NONSENSE HEALTH GUIDE

HOW TO TONE AND TRIM YOUR TROUBLE SPOTS

By the Editors of
Prevention® Magazine

Longmeadow Press

Notice

This book is intended as a reference volume only, not as a medical manual or guide to self-treatment. It is not intended as a substitute for the medical advice of physicians. The reader should regularly consult a physician in general, and particularly for any symptoms. If you suspect that you have a medical problem, we urge you to seek competent medical help. Keep in mind that exercise and nutritional needs vary from person to person, depending on age, sex, health status and individual variations. The information here is intended to help you make informative decisions about your health, not as a substitute for any treatment that may have been prescribed by your doctor.

How to Tone and Trim Your Trouble Spots

Copyright © 1987 Rodale Press, Inc. All Rights Reserved.

Cover Art © 1987 by Rodale Press

Published April 1987 for Longmeadow Press, 201 High Ridge Road, Stamford, CT 06904. No part of this book may be reproduced or used in any form or by any means, electronic or mechanical, including photocopying, recording, or by any information storage and retrieval system, without permission in writing from the publisher.

Library of Congress Cataloging-in-Publication Data

How to tone and trim your trouble spots.

    (No-nonsense health guide)
    1. Exercise.   2. Reducing exercise.   3. Physical fitness.   I. Prevention (Emmaus, Pa.)   II. Series. [DNLM: 1. Exertion—popular works.   2. Physical Fitness—popular works.   QT 260 H847]
GV508.H68   1987   613.7′1   87-2662
ISBN 0-681-40131-1   paperback

Special thanks to Martha Capwell for compiling and editing the information in this book.

Book design by Acey Lee and Lisa Gatti

Photographs by Margaret Skrovanek pp. 5, 6, 12; Christie C. Tito pp. 25, 26, 27, 28.

2 4 6 8 10 9 7 5 3 1   paperback

Contents

Spot Reducing— Can It Be Done?

You've probably spent more than a few minutes lurking around bookstore shelves examining those 30-day spot-exercise books and wondering if they work. They don't, says Bryant Stamford, Ph.D., from the Exercise Physiology Laboratory at the University of Louisville School of Medicine in Kentucky.

"First of all, any book that promises results in a short amount of time, with a minimum of effort, just doesn't work. Anything you do toward fat reduction and fitness is only going to work with a fair amount of effort over an extended period of time," he says. And since those books often emphasize spot exercises, they're ineffective because spot exercises don't work, according to Dr. Stamford.

"There's a popular misconception that when you exercise a specific muscle group, the muscles reach out and grab the surrounding fat and burn it up," he says. But when you exercise a specific area, you're using up fats immobilized all around the body—not just in one spot.

"What's worse, spot exercises usually use fairly small muscle groups and don't burn up a lot of calories. If you're going to lose fat, you've got to burn up a lot of calories."

That is not to say that localized exercises of lesser muscle groups are wasted effort. They *do* burn calories, and they also can provide greater muscle tone to areas that may appear fatter than they actually are simply because of sagging.

Which brings us to toning, the stretching and strengthening of muscle, old or new. Such movement is fundamental in the fitness world, but not everyone realizes just how much toning can do for the human physique.

Ellington Darden, Ph.D., exercise expert and author of *The Nautilus Woman,* points out that stretching and strengthening the right muscles can reduce flabbiness on the buttocks and hips, give greater definition to the thighs and calves, make the shoulders appear broader or less bony, improve the contours of the midsection, enhance erect and confident posture and even give more poise to sagging breasts. And no doubt hundreds of other fitness experts would agree—and add a list of visual benefits of their own. It's simple common sense that by improving the function of muscles, their form naturally improves.

Chapter by chapter, then, we'll guide you through techniques to improve the look and feel of your most persistent trouble spots, keeping in mind the role of *total* body fitness in overall appearance.

Easy Push-Ups for Upper Body Strength

Ah, the Push-Up. From high school gym class to Army training camp to today's exercise and fitness classes, the Push-Up is one calisthenic you can't seem to get away from.

Whether you like it or not, it's a good way to develop upper body strength, especially if you don't have regular access to weight-training equipment. "The Push-Up is similar to a Bench Press," says Michael H. Stone, Ph.D., an exercise physiologist at Auburn University's National Strength Research Center, Auburn, Alabama. "It works the pectorals (chest muscles), deltoids (front shoulder muscles) and triceps (muscles at the back of the upper arm)."

For those of us who haven't lifted our own body weight for quite some time, the Push-Up may be the ideal place to start strengthening the upper body.

Start Simple

But what if the classic Push-Up is a tad too difficult for you right off the bat? Irving Dardik, M.D., an Olympic trainer and coauthor of

1

Quantum Fitness, recommends a series of Push-Ups, from a simple Wall Push-Up through a difficult Chair Push-Up, to help you build up to a very challenging exercise. Do each exercise three times and move to the next one. Build your stamina until you can do the series three times.

1. Wall Push-Up.   Stand a foot or so away from a wall, facing the wall. With your arms extended from your sides and raised to shoulder level, bend your elbows and press your palms against the wall. Keep your abdomen tucked in. Lean into the wall, keeping your body in a straight line from shoulder to heel. If you keep your elbows extended to the sides, you'll be working the pectoral muscles of your chest; if your elbows are at your sides, you will be working your triceps. Continue to keep your abdominals contracted. (Your heels may rise off the floor, which indicates that your back leg muscles aren't very flexible.) Return to the starting position.

2. Chair Push-Up.   This is a somewhat more difficult version of the Wall Push-Up. Place a sturdy, armless chair against a wall, with the seat facing you. Kneel in front of the chair. Place your hands on the sides of the chair seat, toward the front. Keeping your arms straight, walk your legs out behind you until your body is in a straight line. Lower yourself slowly to the chair with your arms. (Keeping your elbows close to your body allows both arm and chest muscles to share the load.) Then raise yourself slowly, still keeping your body in a straight line.

3. Floor Push-Up.   This is the classic Push-Up. Lower yourself to the floor and stretch out in a horizontal position, supporting yourself with your extended arms. Then lower your body to the floor. You can increase the difficulty of the exercise by doing these Push-Ups on closed fists or on your fingertips. Again, if you keep your elbows at your sides, you'll work your arm muscles. If you keep them extended, you'll work your chest muscles.

4. Inverted Chair Push-Up.   This is the most difficult version of the Push-Up. It follows the same basic formula as the preceding variations. Begin by lying on your stomach in front of a chair that's pushed against a wall. Prop your toes on the chair behind you, then raise your body by extending your arms. (The higher the chair, the

more your feet are raised and the more difficult the exercise becomes.)
Be sure to keep your body straight as you lower it.

A final note for women: Push-Ups may be particularly difficult for
you because women generally have less upper body strength than men.
And the easy Push-Ups you may have been taught in school (keeping
the knees on the floor) are practically worthless, because you lift only a
small percentage of your total body weight, according to Dianne Hales
and Lt. Col. Robert E. Hales, M.D., authors of *The U.S. Army Total
Fitness Program.* You can either start with Dr. Dardik's easier Push-
Ups or try the exercise the Hales suggest, called a Negative Push-Up.
Here's how:

Get down on your hands and knees and then into the "up"
Push-Up position. Your arms should be fully extended and your body
straight. Hold this position for several seconds. Then begin lowering
your body, a few inches at a time, holding each position for a few
seconds. Continue lowering your body until your chest is almost on the
floor. When you can't hold it any longer, lower your body onto the floor
and relax. Do as many of these Negative Push-Ups as you can, taking
about 12 seconds for each one. The Hales say that after a while you'll
find you can hold each Push-Up position much longer than before.
When you can, you're ready to try a regular Push-Up, going all the way
down and then pushing all the way back up with your arms.

For more upper body exercises, see chapters 2, 3 and 16.

Building Biceps, Firming Triceps

Want to trade in your soft, wiggly upper arms for firmer, sleeker, better-toned limbs that look great in sleeveless clothing? Working out regularly with light weights provides the resistance your upper arms need to tone and define muscles you didn't know you had. (Women, don't worry that you'll end up looking like a female Rambo. The female body simply doesn't produce enough testosterone and other male hormones that are responsible for the massive upper arms achieved by male body builders.)

Toning and Strengthening Your Upper Arms, Front and Back

For the best visual effect, work both the bicep (the large muscle at the front of the upper arm—the one you can see when you "flex") and the corresponding tricep (the less visible but equally useful large muscle on the back of your upper arm). These easy dumbbell workouts can go a long way to counteract persistent upper arm flab—and build strength as a bonus.

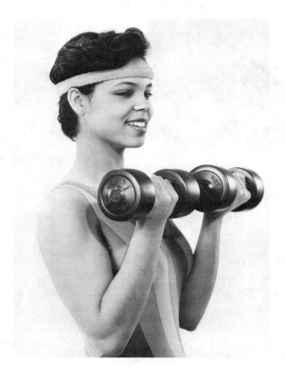

Biceps. Stand erect and hold a dumbbell (five pounds or less) in each hand, with your arms at your sides and your palms facing forward. Slowly bend your arms at the elbows and bring the weights up until they touch your chest. Do ten repetitions.

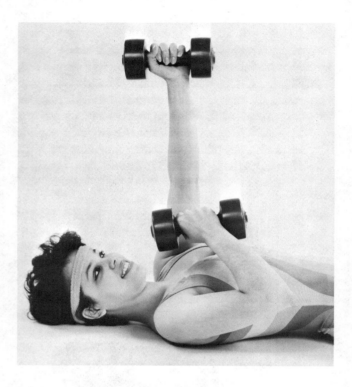

Triceps.   Lie on your back on the floor and hold a pair of dumbbells (five pounds each, or less) directly overhead, with your arms straight. Then slowly lower the weights toward your chest, bending your elbows. You can work both arms simultaneously or one at a time. Do ten repetitions.

For a more elaborate body sculpting routine, refer to chapter 16. The technique works by reducing overall body fat and firming particular muscles to produce stronger lines.

C H A P T E R
T H R E E

Bust Developers— Myths and Facts

"The bigger the better"—that's the way many women feel about their breasts. And if nature doesn't smile on them, they're prepared to go to all ends of the cosmetic counter and figure salon to find happiness.

We decided to follow them—in a manner of speaking.

We started with one of those exercise devices advertised in the back of many women's magazines—you know, the one that resembles a pink plastic clamshell held open by a heavy-duty spring. The idea is to take it in your hands (with your arms extended and flexed in a series of exercise positions) and press against the resistance of the spring to close the shell.

To see the busty, bikini-clad blonde in the instruction manual perform the exercise, it looks like effortless grace. But you almost need Arnold Schwarzenegger to carry it off picture-perfect! The exercises do seem to work on the chest muscles. If you place the palms of your hands together in front of your chest, with your elbows out to the sides, and press your palms together hard, you'll actually feel the muscles across your chest tighten. And if you're somewhat out of shape, ten minutes with one of these devices is liable to leave your chest muscles feeling like your stomach muscles do after 100 Sit-Ups.

You might expect some backing from exercise experts for these devices. But surprisingly, Dorothy V. Harris, Ph.D., a professor of physical education and the director of the Research Center for Women in Sports at Pennsylvania State University, gives them the "thumbs down."

"There's no way exercise will increase mammary tissue," she told us. "In fact, it's a misnomer to say that anything will increase the size of the actual breast."

That's because exercise tends to strengthen and enlarge muscle mass. Since the breasts consist of fatty and glandular tissue—no muscle—there's nothing there to build up.

The chest muscles, or pectorals, on the other hand, may benefit from a daily workout, but not to the extent that most women would hope, Dr. Harris explains.

"Thanks to Mother Nature and hormone levels, females just do not have the same predisposition to muscle bulking that males do," she insists. "A high testosterone [male hormone] level is needed to increase muscle girth. That's why the average woman can pump iron regularly and experience only a minimal increase in chest size."

Proof of this comes from Jack H. Wilmore, Ph.D., professor and head of the department of physical education at the University of Arizona, Tucson.

In the *Journal of Sports Medicine,* Dr. Wilmore writes that he put 47 women and 26 men through an identical weight-training program. The group worked out twice a week, 40 minutes a day, for a total of ten weeks. During that time, both the men and the women increased the strength of their upper body. But, he reports, there was very little increase in the muscle bulk of the women participants.

Well then, what about firming and toning sagging breast tissue?

"No exercise in the world will regain the elasticity of the breast once it's lost," Dr. Harris sighs. That's because there are no muscles in the breasts, only two ligaments—called Cooper's ligaments—which keep the breasts tilted upward. But once they've stretched, you've got "Cooper's droop," and there's not too much you can do to reverse it. "Better to prevent it before it happens by providing adequate support—especially during physical activity," Dr. Harris suggests. (For more information on preventing breasts from sagging, see "Boosting Your Bust," later in this chapter.)

The Protein Ploy

Protein for the bust is another advertising ploy that seems to have little merit. Granted, good nutrition is essential to a healthy body. And when your body is alive with good health, it radiates in the way you look.

But as Gideon G. Panter, M.D., a New York City gynecologist and a faculty member at New York Hospital–Cornell Medical Center, says, "To suggest that there is one food that goes directly to the breast is absolutely ridiculous!

"The only thing that determines the size of a woman's breasts is genetics. That and the amount of weight she carries. Certainly, if she eats more, she will eventually increase the fat deposits in her breasts. But then she'll be getting heavier all over, not just in one area."

Dr. Panter also disagrees with the idea that a flat-chested woman may be protein deficient and may need a protein supplement to increase muscle and body tone. "Protein deficiency indicates malnutrition," he says. "And that's going to show up with more serious symptoms than a flat chest."

What about Massage and Hormones?

Massage has also been touted as an aid to bust development. We sent for two massage devices. One was described as a "power-packed electric bust-builder" and promised to "melt away fat as it builds up your bust." (It's hard to imagine how they intend to do that!)

The other was called a Hydro-Stimulator, which turned out to be a rather bizarre contraption that hooks up to your water faucet at one end and encases your breast in a blue cup (size 52D) at the other. By producing a whirl of water pressure around the breast, this device supposedly increases circulation and stimulates breast growth.

We asked Dr. Panter if there is anything to this notion. "For sure, stimulation does increase the size of the breasts," he concedes. "Masters and Johnson monitored the breast during preorgasmic stimulation and found that it enlarges by 20 percent."

But don't get your hopes up—it's not what you think. Dr. Panter further explained that the effect does not involve permanent growth but rather temporary swelling. The breasts return to their original size shortly after stimulation.

Can creams increase the size or improve the appearance of the breasts? "That's a Madison Avenue concept!" says Dr. Panter. "You can't change the composition of the skin by smearing it with a greasy cream. Any alteration in skin texture must come from within." For example, estrogen levels seem to be an important influence on a woman's skin—and breast size, for that matter.

Every authority we consulted agreed that estrogen can increase breast size when taken by mouth—as was the case years ago with women on the Pill, before the dosage was decreased due to evidence that high doses were linked to cancer in some women. But there was quite a bit of discrepancy over its effectiveness when mingled with a cream base and rubbed into the skin.

We asked Gary Stein, M.D., epidemiology intelligence service officer for the Centers for Disease Control in Atlanta, whether estrogen can penetrate the skin and enter the bloodstream. He has good reason to believe that you don't necessarily have to take estrogen orally to have it enter your bloodstream.

Dr. Stein took part in a study in Puerto Rico where employees of an Ortho Pharmaceutical Company plant were developing high blood levels of estrogen. The employees affected were involved with the manufacture of birth control pills.

Five out of 25 men who worked in this division showed symptoms of an increase in the female sex hormone and 3 actually developed enlarged breasts. Among the women employees, 2 of the 5 who came in contact with the powdered birth control substance and 10 of 18 in the production line, who worked with the finished product, experienced unusual vaginal bleeding.

How can this phenomenon be explained? "I doubt very much whether there was any direct ingestion of the substance," Dr. Stein says. "But there's a good possibility that skin contact and breathing the airborne particles caused the high estrogen levels in these workers."

Of course, some physicians may argue that there's a difference between powdered estrogen and the estrogen tied up in a cream. So we again asked Dr. Stein if he thought that mattered. "Not really," he replied. "It is still a lipid-soluble-type compound. It can still be absorbed as a cream."

At best, it seems, estrogen creams will produce no results. At worst, they could expose their users to all the possible risks of oral estrogen.

So what's a woman genuinely concerned about her breast size to do? "There's always plastic surgery," Dr. Panter says lightly. "But," he adds, "that's not without considerable risk. It's safer—and cheaper—to pick up a copy of *Vogue* magazine and realize that it's very fashionable these days to be small-chested. Otherwise the only thing that will increase actual breast size is pregnancy. And to minimize sagging and improve tone, try breastfeeding."

Unfortunately, many modern women deny themselves the satisfaction of breastfeeding their children for fear of losing what some consider their "feminine charms." Actually, it may improve their figure.

"Even if you haven't breastfed your first child, breastfeeding the second will help you regain the tone you may have lost during the first pregnancy," Dr. Panter explains. Just be sure to wear a good support bra during the nursing period—even while you're sleeping.

And if you're too old—or too young—for that, remember that body *proportion* is a hundred times more important to your total image than the size and shape of your breasts. So keep in shape with a good physical activity like swimming or jogging. It will improve your posture and get your whole body glowing.

Boosting Your Bust

These exercises—actually variations on one theme, using increasing amounts of weight—tone up your pectoral muscles (the ones that provide the foundation for the bust) and thus help keep your breasts from sagging as much as is physically possible without resorting to surgery. Push-Ups (see chapter 1) will help, too.

1. Lie on the floor with your arms straight out from your shoulders and your palms up. Slowly bring your arms up, keeping your elbows straight, so that they meet in midair above your chest. Cross them lightly forward and then back and then lower them again to the starting position. Repeat 7 times and work up to 16 times.

When you've built up some strength, try doing this exercise

holding a lightweight object in each hand, perhaps two hard-cooked eggs to start, and progressing to increasingly heavy, yet safe and manageable, weights such as rocks or cans.

2. Find two books or other objects of equal weight (but not too heavy!), making sure that you can grasp them easily. Lying flat on the floor with your knees bent, hold the books directly above your head (straight up along your ears, with your arms extended) and slowly raise them toward the ceiling until your arms are extended straight above your chest. Slowly lower the weights, returning them to the floor above your head. Raise again slowly 4 times and gradually increase the number of lifts to 16.

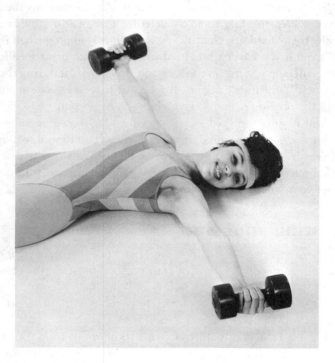

3. Lie on your back on the floor and hold a dumbbell (five pounds or less) in each hand. Hold the dumbbells directly over your chest with your arms straight and your palms facing each other. Then, keeping your arms straight, slowly lower the weights to the floor on each side so

your body forms a cross. Then bring the weights to the upright position again. Do 10 repetitions and gradually work up to 20.

Swimming is another great bust toner, especially the aptly named breast stroke. To make your arms and chest do all the work, don't kick. Anchor your legs with a Styrofoam pull buoy to keep your lower half from sinking. For a real upper body workout, add about a pound of ankle weights.

These exercises, along with the ones in chapters 1 and 2, will help bring about a more upwardly beautiful you.

Declare War against Those Love Handles

If a guy can take a pinch of flesh at his sides just above his beltline and not regret the amount that he comes up with, he's one very rare American male. Even some avid runners want to know what to do about their accursed "love handles."

Well, the answer is not an easy one, because love handles exist not solely due to sloth. They exist due to genetic predisposition, which means that if you have love handles, your granddad probably did, too. (Men, for reasons not yet fully understood, simply tend to put weight on first—and lose it last—from the area around the midsection. Women, by comparison, tend to collect excess poundage around the hips, thighs and upper arms.)

Despite their genesis, love handles can be lost. The loss is not apt to be easy, and you may find yourself losing weight around the neck and face first, but be patient. The love handles *will* go.

A Three-Pronged Attack

We've put together a weight-loss program with copious abdomens specifically in mind. It's a three-pronged attack that involves eating less, exercising more and doing specific exercises for toning the muscles at your sagging midsection.

But wouldn't just one of these approaches be enough, you ask? Probably not. Dieting, certainly, would bring about some improvement in time. But without exercise, there would be loss of muscle tissue in addition to loss of fat. And your midsection, as you may have guessed, is encumbered primarily by the latter.

What about just stepping up your overall exercise program?

Again, you might see some improvement, but it would be slow. And unless your program included specific exercises for tightening the muscles beneath your abdominal flesh, you would be doing little to reduce the amount of sag that is at the core of that love-handle look.

So what about just doing Sit-Ups until you're blue in the face?

If you could do enough of them to burn a significant number of calories, you might make some headway. But, as evidenced by an experiment done by Frank Katch, Ed.D., at the University of Massachusetts, that would have to be quite a lot. Fifteen people were made to do Sit-Ups five days a week for 5½ weeks. And even after progressing to 336 a day (having started out at 70 a day), they experienced no reduction in waist size or amount of abdominal fat. So much for Sit-Ups. (They're good, if done properly, for toning the muscles *beneath* excess flesh, but they do nothing to help burn abdominal fat in a localized way. "Spot reducing" is just not in the cards.)

And what about sauna belts?

Any reduction a sauna belt produces is the result of temporary (and we emphasize temporary) dehydration of tissue in the area where it is worn. A couple of Perriers and you're back out to where you belong.

There is, in a word, no easy way. Love handles demand all-out war. And if you're willing to declare that war, here is your best plan of attack.

Moderate reduction of caloric intake.   By moderate we mean something between 200 and 500 calories a day. You can do it any way you like, but it would be our suggestion that you cut down on fatty condiments (butter, mayonnaise, salad oils, sour cream and the like), alcohol and sugar.

Moderate increase in levels of physical activity.   If you're already in command of a fitness routine you're proud of, this need not apply to you. But if you know that you're spending more time sitting around than you should, make some changes. They don't have to be major ones, but they *should* be daily. Things like taking the stairs instead of the elevator and using your push mower this summer more often than your riding mower. Exercise doesn't have to happen in a sweat suit in order to burn calories.

Specific exercises (done at least five days a week) for toning the muscles beneath your chunky middle.

The muscles of the abdomen are a little like a tire—layered, in two plies. And in order to firm up the entire package, it's best to do a separate exercise for each.

A word on Straight-Leg Sit-Ups (and Leg Lifts): They may feel as though they're getting to your abdomen, but Sit-Ups and Leg Lifts done with the legs straight actually give more of a workout to muscles of the lower back and thighs. Therefore, you should do Sit-Ups *with your legs bent,* such as these manuevers:

1. Lie on your back, bend your knees and rest your calves on a box or footstool. Curl into a tuck position, hold for several seconds, and return to the floor. Do only as many as feel comfortable in the beginning (3 to 10) but feel free to build up to 100 or so.

2. Lying on your back with your arms outstretched, hold your knees and ankles together and draw your legs up to your chest. Then simply flop your legs (slowly) back and forth from one side of your body to the other. Again, 10 or so should feel like a workout in the beginning, but 50 to 100 should not be out of order within several months.

3. Lie on the floor and prepare to do a Bent-Leg Sit-Up. Cross your arms over your chest. With each Sit-Up, twist your torso and swing your right elbow to your left side, then your left elbow to your right side. As with the other exercises, start with about ten, and progress as you see fit. This exercise works the front and sides of your abdomen.

The Logic behind Our Love-Handle Attack

By reducing calories an average of 300 a day and stepping up caloric expenditures by an average of 200 a day (your stomach exercises alone should be worth about 100), you put yourself on the good side of 500 calories daily, which, multiplied by seven days, equals 3,500 calories a week—the equivalent of one pound of fat. Over a two-month period, that comes to eight pounds—a sizable dent in anybody's middle.

Whittle Your Waist

The popular expression is "flatten your stomach," but a flabby paunch really has nothing to do with the condition of your stomach, which is a digestive organ, not a muscle. What you really need to work on are your abdominals (abs, for short), a muscle group consisting of four major muscles.

- The rectus muscle, the strongest of the group, runs vertically down the center of your body from midribs to the pelvis. The rectus muscle controls the tilt of the pelvis and, consequently, the curvature of the spine.
- The transverse muscle, in the lower part of the abdomen, reaches around both sides of your body, under and perpendicular to the rectus muscle. It helps hold your abdomen flat when it's toned.
- The internal and external oblique muscles are two layers of muscles that run diagonally in opposite directions from the hipbones toward the ribs, interlacing with the transverse muscle. The obliques are vital for a trim waistline.

No other part of the body is quite as troublesome as the abdomen when it comes to getting in shape and looking good. But looking good is only one reason to tone your abs. A well-toned abdominal wall is also critical for good posture and a healthy back. (See chapter 14 for more about keeping your back in shape.)

Unfortunately, most popular sports, like jogging, bicycling and tennis, don't work to tone the abdominal muscles. As one sports medicine expert put it, "The only time during the day you use your abdominal muscles directly is when you sit up in bed." That isn't enough exercise to strengthen them.

Since the sole support of your lower back is your abdominal wall, drooping abdominal muscles can make you more susceptible to one of the most common afflictions of humankind—the aching back. The muscles that form your abdominal wall actually prevent the spine from falling forward.

It might seem hard to believe, but when you're standing, the load on your back is more than half your total body weight. Normal everyday activities, like sitting, can increase that load on the lower back to several times your body weight.

"About 80 percent of all lower back disorders originate from the musculature," says Charles Dotson, Ph.D., professor of physical education at the University of Maryland. Weak abdominal muscles shift the body's center of gravity forward, so the back compensates by increasing the curvature of the spine. "The back muscles work to maintain poor posture and become fatigued," Dr. Dotson says. Improper spinal alignment can cause the links of the spine, the intervertebral disks, to compress. Gradually, the disk herniates, or "slips," and rubs painfully against nerves in the back. You can prevent or reduce the risk of a herniated disk and other back problems by exercising your abdominal muscles.

"Stomach Fat"—
The First to Arrive, the Last to Go

If your main concern is toning and trimming, keep in mind that spot reducing is a fallacy. "To a certain extent, you can tone the muscles of a particular region, but there is no such thing as causing fat to leave that region," says Dr. Dotson. What's frustrating, he adds, is that the abdomen is the first place most people deposit fat. And it's the very last and most difficult area from which to get rid of fat. "You can do a million Sit-Ups, but if you haven't lost body fat, you'll still have a belly," says one sports physiologist. The solution: Lose fat by exercising and changing eating habits, and tone muscle by exercising.

The Best Workout

These exercises help correct physical faults over time as well as improve your flexibility. As you do them, concentrate on your abdominal muscles and your breathing. Move smoothly and gradually. Relax, keeping enough tone and control to hold the position.

Pelvic Tilt. This exercise will familiarize you with your lower back and abdominal muscles. To start, lie on the floor with your arms at your sides and your palms down. Your spine is almost flat against the floor and your chin is pressed toward your chest. Your legs are straight and parallel and your feet are fully stretched. Tense your thigh muscles, but don't lock your knees. Put your hand in the space between your lower back and the floor. Press your navel to your spine and your spine to the floor. The space around your hand should decrease. Relax and take your hand out from behind your back. Repeat the movement and see if you feel the same muscles working.

Roll-Up. Start in the same position as for the Pelvic Tilt. Breathe in and roll up for 12 counts, vertebra by vertebra. Press your chin toward your chest as you bring your head off the floor. Look at your abdomen; the abdominal muscles should be flattened, not puffed out.

Your arms will naturally slide forward along the floor. When your forehead is near your knees, breathe out and reach forward to elongate your spine. Don't tilt your head up; reach forward with a straight spine. Now breathe out and roll down in eight counts.

Hip Roll. This exercise uses the transverse muscle. Lie on the floor with your arms extended out from your shoulders and your palms flat on the floor. Bring your knees toward your chest, with your feet close to your buttocks. Your entire spine should be flat on the floor.

Roll onto your right buttock, keeping your shoulders anchored to the floor and your feet close to your buttocks. When you roll to the right, your left shoulder may start to come off the floor, but don't let it. Roll back to the starting position, then repeat to the other side.

Leg Lower. Leg Lowers work the lower part of the rectus muscle, a real trouble spot. Lie flat on your back with your arms out to the sides. Press your chin toward your chest and look at your abdomen. Draw your knees toward your chest and unfold your legs so they're perpendicular to the floor. Lower your legs only as far as you can while keeping your lower back on the floor. Find the point that's right for you. Hold for five counts. Bend your legs and bring them back toward your chest. Repeat. The farther down your legs can go, the stronger your abdominal muscles are.

Cat Curl. This will increase suppleness in your lower back. Move slowly! Get on your hands and knees, placing your hands directly below your shoulders with your arms rotated in so your fingertips face each other. Keep your legs hip-width apart, with your knees directly below the hip sockets. Start with an indented lower back, keeping your head facing forward. Beginning at the base of the spine, press your abdominal wall toward your lower back, gradually rounding your spine.

Imagine there's a weight pressing down on your lower back, and try to push it up. Now the weight overpowers you and causes your lower back to indent first, then slowly indents your entire back.

Sit-Up. Although Sit-Ups are the classic abdominal exercises, most people do them incorrectly. As explained in chapter 4, Straight-Leg Sit-Ups are passé and potentially dangerous. Bent-Leg Sit-Ups are much better for your back. But too many people come all the way up, says Michael Wolf, Ph.D., an independent sports scientist and author. "Coming all the way up is a 50 percent waste of time," he says.

And many people still don't understand that anchoring your feet is also a Sit-Up no-no, says Marilyn I. Miller of San Francisco, who is a registered physical therapist and back-care consultant to business and industry. Anchoring your feet during a Sit-Up (having your feet held down or hooked under something) defeats the purpose of the exercise—which is to use your abdominal muscles.

Instead of using your abdominals, doing a Sit-Up with your feet anchored forces you to depend on your legs and your iliopsoas, a complex of muscles in the hip area, says Miller. The iliopsoas affects the entire working of the back, hips and pelvis.

To make matters worse, in most people the iliopsoas complex is already too tight—it needs to be stretched. But doing a Sit-Up with the feet anchored just tightens it even more. And that can lead to back problems and other related aches and pains.

Anchoring your feet underneath something can also force your body toward a swayback, a vulnerable back and posture position many of us already use in everyday life. Doing Sit-Ups in this weakened position can even *cause* back injury, Miller says.

To do a Sit-Up properly, sit on the floor with your knees bent, but don't anchor your feet. Cross your arms on your chest and slowly curl up halfway. Hold for five counts, release, then repeat.

Tips for Beginners

If your feet tend to fly into the air when you try to do Sit-Ups without anchoring your feet, you can retrain your muscles by doing Curl-Backs and Curl-Ups.

Curl-Back.   Begin a Curl-Back by sitting on the floor with your knees bent, your back rounded and your arms stretched out in front of you. As you pull your navel (or lower abdomen) back and up toward your spine, bend your head forward, focusing on your navel.

Curl slowly back toward the floor, keeping your trunk curled and your head down. Breathe out as you curl back, since this helps you to further contract your abdominals. When you reach the floor, stretch your arms out behind you, unbend your head and take a deep breath.

The object of this exercise is to curl back as slowly as possible while your heels remain in contact with the floor. Once you can do the Curl-Back evenly in a smooth and continuous motion that lasts at least five seconds, you're ready to try a Curl-Up.

Curl-Up.   This is the reverse of the Curl-Back. Lie flat on the floor with your knees bent and your arms stretched out on the floor above your head. Then stretch your arms up over your head and forward. Suck in your abdominals, breathe out and smoothly curl yourself up into a sitting position. Keep your back rounded and your head down and focused on your navel. If you can't do this at first without your feet flying up, try placing your feet *over* an anchor bar, such as those found in many gyms.

Once you can do the Curl-Up without your feet coming off the floor, you can perform both exercises in one continuous sequence. Remember to breathe out as you curl back, then inhale, exhaling again as you curl up. As it becomes easier to sit up, challenge yourself by placing your hands across your chest.

Chapters 4, 14 and 15 offer some more tips for minimizing your midsection.

Fighting Desk-Worker's Spread

Anyone who works at a desk job and doesn't get much exercise worries about a saggy bottom—a spreading posterior that can make shopping for pants or skirts an ordeal. The suit jacket fits, but the pants have to be let out in the seat. The skirt fits at the waist, but it's too tight in the rear.

So what's a saggy bottom to do? You've probably guessed by now—aerobic exercise. Any type should do the trick: swimming, walking, running, jogging or others, says Bryant Stamford, Ph.D., of the Exercise Physiology Laboratory at the University of Louisville School of Medicine in Kentucky. "Aerobic exercises strengthen the big muscle groups, and they're calorie burners. That will have a big impact on fat."

Tightening Your Tush

While you are shedding your excess rear-end baggage, you can tone and define the muscles of your hips and thighs with this modified Squat. Start with a fairly light weight and build up to a heavier one.

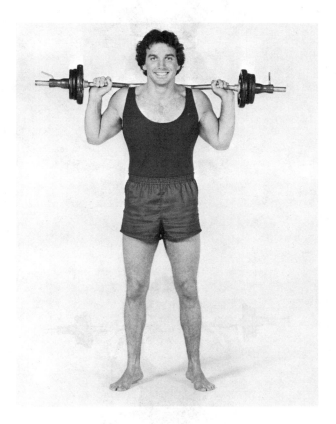

Stand with your feet slightly more than shoulder-width apart, with your toes angled outward. Hold a barbell across your shoulders and slowly bend your knees until your thighs are parallel to the floor. Then return to the erect position. Do 10 to 12 repetitions, and use enough weight to make the tenth repetition a tough one.

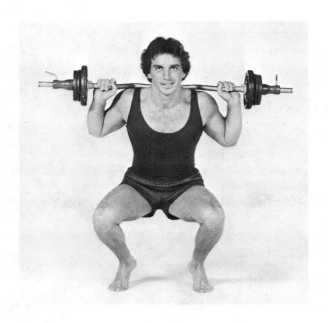

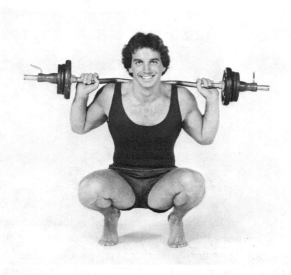

Pick a focal point for your eyes during the exercise and keep your eyes on that point the whole time. This will help keep your body in the proper upright position and put less stress on your lower back.

An important point to remember about Squats is not to bounce on your way down. Bouncing puts tremendous pressure on your knees and may cause joint problems that will outweigh the exercise's benefits.

Lunges are also a good way to slim down leg and rear-end fat. They are similar to Squats. The weights are held with the barbell across your shoulders, but your feet are separated, with one foot forward and the

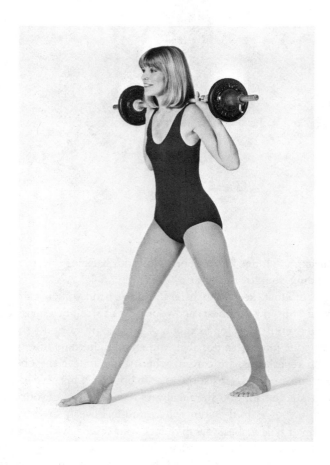

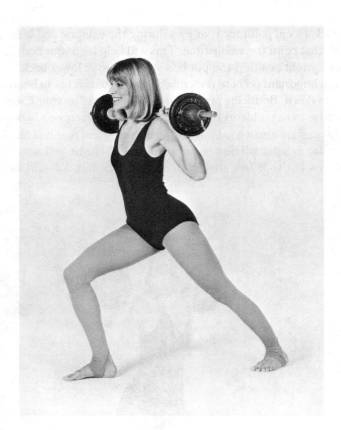

other back. You lunge forward, bringing your back leg toward the floor and bending your front leg at a 90-degree angle. Again, as you did during the Squat, keep your head up (don't bend your neck down or bury your chin in your chest) and your back as straight as possible. To make the exercise develop as much of a range of motion—the movement of your joints—as possible, you should alternate foot positions every ten repetitions. Be careful when you get near the end of the exercise and are tired—resist the urge to bounce. This urge gets worse when fatigue sets in. You should always retain control of your body, so quit before you get to the point where you feel overly tired.

Chapter 8 describes ways to reduce your thighs, which are usually part of that desk-worker's saggy baggage, too. And you think you have a cellulite problem? You don't. Read the next chapter to find out why.

C H A P T E R
S E V E N

The Plain Truth about Cellulite

It's the dimpled and puckered flab that clings to thighs, buttocks, arms and hips—called orange-peel skin by some, cottage-cheese fat by others and cellulite by most. But whatever it's called, cellulite is widely regarded as one of the toughest of all physical blemishes to erase. It's said to afflict eight out of ten women (and a few men) and is the bane of the beauty-conscious.

Popular lore says that cellulite (a term coined in European salons and spas) is not ordinary fat but "fat gone wrong," a gel-like blend of fat, water and toxins pocketed in tiny lumps just beneath the skin. Press your skin between your hands, some people advise, and you'll probably see the oatmeal lumps of cellulite. For such deformity they blame birth control pills, internal illnesses, environmental pollutants and even—would you believe—miniskirts.

According to a few self-styled experts, getting rid of cellulite is not like getting rid of ordinary fat. Simple dieting and exercise, they say, won't work on this pseudofat. Effective treatment calls for unusual—even bizarre—approaches. Thus, the "cures" have included loofah

Thin Thighs from a Bottle?

The anticellulite creams may sport French-sounding trade names, contain everything from sea moss to horse chestnuts and boast the power to kill cellulite where it sits. The manufacturers say that the creams can "contour" the body, "tone superficial tissues" and offer "sleekening benefits."

But, alas, the ballyhoo is bunk. A U.S. Food and Drug Administration report points out that despite their exotic contents, the creams include the same types of ingredients as common lubricating lotions: water, emollients, emulsifiers, preservatives, colors and fragrances. And experts have already insisted there isn't a shred of medical evidence that the creams work.

sponges, cactus-fiber washcloths, horsehair mitts, vitamin/mineral supplements, rubberized pants, toning lotions, creams, enzyme injections, vibrating machines and whirlpool baths.

Unfortunately, none of these miracles works. And for good reason. Doctors and researchers point out that cellulite is not "fat gone wrong"—it's just plain fat. Scientists can detect no chemical or structural difference between so-called cellulite fat and common fat. The disorder, therefore, will respond to dieting and exercise, but not to the offbeat remedies that have nothing to do with fat reduction.

Researchers now know that what people call cellulite is simply ordinary fat cells overloaded with fat and bulging underneath the skin in a waffled pattern. "What you see is a combination of fat, poor muscle tone and poor skin tone," says Neil Solomon, M.D., an obesity and weight-control expert in Baltimore. "It's the way the skin fits over whatever fat there is underneath. If a person does not have good muscle tone in an area, say on the thighs, the skin takes on the contours of the fat beneath and appears rippled."

Researchers also know that some people are more prone to the condition than others, and the reasons are sex and heredity. A pair of

German investigators found that women are more likely than men to have cellulite partly because the fat just beneath women's skin is packed into round fat-cell chambers that can easily bulge underneath the skin, while men's fat-cell chambers are arranged in a more stable design. And perhaps just as important, certain areas of women's skin are actually thinner than men's and have more fat under the surface. Then, too, people vary greatly in their patterns of fat distribution, and children are likely to inherit the patterns of their parents.

Two Ways to Get Rid of Cellulite

But these givens of gender and heredity can be improved upon, and medical professionals say there are only two ways to do it: You have to consistently take in fewer calories than you expend, and you must exercise regularly to tighten up the muscles and make the flabby areas appear taut.

Dr. Solomon emphasizes that in his own studies of weight loss in overweight people with dimpling of the skin on their thighs and buttocks, "those who lost weight lost some of the dimpling."

The German researchers concur with Dr. Solomon and underscore the importance of physical activity in the battle against cellulite. They claim, as other researchers do, that they've seen little or no cellulite among female athletes.

Running, dancing, swimming, cycling—these and other activities can help you burn off flab, but some fitness experts say that one of the best anticellulite exercises is walking. For walking helps pull on—and thus firm—buttocks and thighs, areas most susceptible to "orange-peel skin."

Dr. Solomon does, however, offer a caution to those who try to lose too much too fast: "Don't lose more weight (not more than five to ten pounds a month) than your skin elasticity can keep up with. In an older person, bat-wing arms and wrinkled, flabby skin on the abdomen are usually the results of too-rapid weight loss and insufficient regular exercise."

(For more on trimming away fat from your thighs, see the next chapter.)

A Whole-Body Approach to Thinner Thighs

What is it with thighs? Why are they such trouble spots for women?

As mentioned elsewhere in this book, women have a hormonal predisposition to accumulate fat on the breasts, buttocks, hips and thighs. Heredity dictates where the greatest concentrations will be (not all of us can be a perfect size eight). And, of course, the older we get, the more fat we tend to store. But it is possible to prevent yourself from becoming too bottom heavy by watching your weight and getting plenty of exercise. If you're careful not to put on too much weight, there won't be any fat to accumulate—no matter what your genes hold in store for you.

The best type of exercise for reducing the girth of the hips and thighs without overly increasing muscle mass is aerobic exercise. That is, walking, running, cycling, swimming and the like. A regular, vigorous program incorporating one or more of such activities increases our ability to burn fat stores as fuel. And in most cases, the fat that's first to go (the body does not discriminate) will be in the area of greatest concentration. If that's your hips, thighs or buttocks, then you're on your way.

It's important to keep in mind that there is a difference between spot reducing (trying to burn fat in a specific area by exercising a specific muscle group) and spot toning. It is possible to tone up the muscles of the thighs through specific exercises—such as Side Leg Lifts. Lie on your side on the floor, with your legs straight and your elbow supporting your upper body. Point the toe of your upper leg and lift your leg as high as you can. Lower, then repeat ten times. Turn on your other side and repeat ten more times.

Here's another good thigh toner: Stand about a foot away from a wall and lean back so your shoulders and back touch the wall, then slide your back down the wall until your knees are bent and your thighs are parallel to the floor. Hold for as long as you can. Each day, gradually increase the holding time. This exercise tones but, again, it will not reduce excess fat.

The exercises for a sagging seat in chapter 6 will firm up your thighs, too.

Losing the Ten Pounds Winter Left Behind

"April is the cruelest month," goes the famous line from T. S. Eliot's poem *The Waste Land.* Maybe that poem should have been called *The Waist Land,* because April *is* the cruelest month for those of us who manage to put on five or ten pounds every winter. What's more cruel than spring clothes that feel like they shrank mysteriously? Just the thought of summer beaches and bathing suits is enough to make you grimace.

So rather than cover them up with a jacket, get rid of those extra pounds. The way to start, of course, is by stepping up your exercise program. Luckily, the weather should dovetail nicely with your renewed efforts. But if you're already exercising and the pounds don't seem to come off, it may be time to alter your eating lifestyle.

Notice that we didn't say it's time to "diet." It's pretty much an accepted fact in the world of weight-watching that most so-called diets are quick-fix solutions that almost guarantee you'll gain the weight back when you go "off" the diet.

What most weight-loss counselors now advise is that you change the eating habits that put the pounds on—and thus take them off for good. Although their advice is usually tailored to the very overweight, many of their tips and ideas for changing habits can easily be adapted for people with only minor weight problems. Here's how.

Where Those Pounds Came From

You wouldn't begin a new business venture without first educating yourself about the area you're entering. The same should be true here. You don't have to cut out any basic food to lose weight—you just need to learn about the foods you eat.

Carol Caldwell, a dietitian who advises executives at Canyon Ranch Spa's executive renewal program in Tucson, Arizona, says she gives her clients two basic rules. The first: Don't add fat to fat. "By that I mean when something has been cooked with fat, like a waffle or a muffin, don't add a fat like butter or margarine to it." What, then, do you spread on? "Try jam instead. Yes, it has sugar, but it has many fewer calories, and you tend to use less of it than butter," says Caldwell.

Caldwell's second rule is: Don't add protein to protein. "For example, when you order a chef's salad, it usually has four protein foods— ham, cheese, egg and turkey. Ask the chef to leave off all but one protein food, preferably the turkey because it's lowest in fat.

"Another good example is pizza. It's really not so bad in calories if you leave off the sausage and pepperoni and instead order it with vegetables like mushrooms, green peppers and onions."

Caldwell says you can continue to eat almost any food you like, with a few alterations. "If you like to snack on cheese and crackers, just eat more crackers than cheese. If you're used to potato chips, switch over to pretzels, which have a lot fewer calories.

"Don't think you have to give up sandwiches if you're trying to cut back. Just avoid the salads, like tuna, egg and chicken, and go for plain meats like turkey and roast beef. And use mustard instead of mayonnaise for a dressing."

Caldwell says gourmet mustards flavored with wines and different spices are great substitute toppings for potatoes. She also advises executives to go ahead and eat pasta—just go for tomato sauces with fish or vegetables rather than cream sauces such as that on fettuccine Alfredo.

The Executive's Guide to Low-Calorie Lunches

The executive lunch—is it a high-calorie trap unavoidable by those in the business world? Well, the lunch may be unavoidable, but the high calories aren't.

Dining out lightly in restaurants is a challenge for the weight-conscious. Here's what the experts recommend:

- Frequent the same restaurants so that the waiters and waitresses get to know you. They'll make it a habit to leave the rolls off the table, and they'll remember other weight-watchers' requests.
- Decide before you get to the restaurant what you're going to have. If broiled fish is what you've decided on, you won't even need to look at the menu—just ask what

Discover Your Food Cues

Becoming educated about foods is just the first step. Next you may want to modify your behavior when it comes to eating. Experts in the weight-loss field have had their greatest successes with very overweight people when they teach them to change their behavior around food.

One of the best ways to do that is to discover what spurs you to eat—what the experts call food cues. The most obvious one for most people is the refrigerator. Just looking at it sets off a desire to eat. How to fight off the urge? Well, you may have to enlist your family's help, but the best thing you can do is get the tempting foods out of sight—in the back of shelves or drawers or stashed away in the freezer. Keep low-calorie foods or things you're not likely to grab, like eggs and butter, toward the front.

You can handle other food cues with other forms of manipulation. If social occasions are your downfall, stay on the other side of the room from the buffet table. Also try to eat something before you go—your will power will get a big boost if you're not starving when you arrive.

kinds they have. Menu reading is one of the biggest traps weight watchers need to avoid.

- If you must look at the menu, scan it quickly and head straight for the "From the Broiler" section or the poultry and fish entrees.
- Ask for sauces and dressings on the side. Or better still, substitute lemon or herbs for the dressings.
- Select a food that must be eaten slowly, like crab legs.
- Order a seltzer water or club soda with lime before lunch. Save the glass of wine for during the meal.
- Frequent Mexican and Italian restaurants. In a survey of popular ethnic restaurants, those two cuisines came out tops in the low-calorie department. Of course, you may want to avoid the garlic and hot chilis if you have any important meetings after lunch!

Slow Down

Another behavior you may want to modify is how fast you eat. Experts believe eating slowly is associated with eating less. Since most of us on busy schedules probably don't take the time to eat slowly, that's a behavior worth tackling. How? Try savoring your food. If you really enjoy eating, chances are you won't rush. Or if you're eating with other people, try this tactic: Don't start until everyone else has begun to eat, and don't be afraid to stop when you've had your fill. "Talk, rearrange your napkin, cut your meat into tiny pieces . . . stall any way you can to be the last person to start eating," says Kelly Brownell, Ph.D., a behavior specialist at the University of Pennsylvania.

Plan Ahead

And finally, think about what you're going to eat. Sure, that'll take some time and effort, but it will keep you from eating things you really don't need. Some experts blame unplanned eating for many cases of overweight. Gerard Musante, Ph.D., a behavioral psychologist who runs Structure House, a weight-loss clinic in Durham, North Carolina, says many people eat out of habit, boredom or stress, without really thinking about what they are doing.

So think ahead before your workday—if you plan to eat only a small lunch and bring fruit to eat during coffee breaks, you're less likely to mindlessly fall prey to glazed doughnuts and Reuben sandwiches. And by the way, if you occasionally decide you do want the Reuben, that's okay, says Dr. Musante—as long as you are aware that you're veering from your plan.

Week-to-Week Success

One final thought about losing weight—the key to success is to go slowly. Nutrition experts say you shouldn't plan to lose more than two pounds a week. Why? Because drastically cutting calories sends a signal to your body to slow down your metabolic rate, which will reduce your ability to burn off fat. It's your body's response to starvation.

So plan to cut back just 500 calories a day if you want to lose about a pound a week. All that means is forgoing your morning pastry at the office and making a few other calorie savings, such as the ones we've described, to be comfortably back in your warm-weather clothes and bathing suit by the end of June.

Preventing– and Erasing– Varicose Veins

Not many conditions can make a person look as old as varicose veins. And the itching, burning and aching can be enough to bring thoughts of early retirement.

And yet, as unpleasant as varicose veins are, they are not uncommon: One out of four women suffers from them, as does one out of ten men.

Why so many?

The tendency to develop varicose veins appears to be inherited, the experts say. But there appear also to be some "aggravating factors," says Howard C. Baron, M.D., a vascular surgeon and author of *Varicose Veins: A Commonsense Approach to Their Management.* "There must be an aggravating factor in lifestyle for the problem to develop. If we avoid aggravating factors, the problem might be delayed or blunted."

A Three-Point Strategy against Varicose Veins

What a varicose vein boils down to is a vein that has lost its ability to move blood along as it should.

But, you ask, isn't moving blood along the heart's job?

Not entirely. Inside your veins (the blood vessels responsible for transporting blood *back* to the heart) are tiny valves that must be able to close between beats of the heart to prevent blood from seeping backward. When these valves cease to function or begin to leak, you've got pooling of blood—particularly in the lower legs, thanks to gravity. And with pooling of blood come the swollen, distorted and aching veins that doctors call varicose. This pooling of blood, however, can be discouraged by way of regular muscular activity.

1. Flex your muscles.   The muscles of the leg have the potential to serve as "a second heart," says Dr. Baron. When leg muscles contract, they squeeze on the veins, helping move blood along. For this reason, standing or sitting for long periods of time (particularly with your legs crossed, which impedes circulation) can be a vein's worst enemy.

So, tip number one for avoiding varicose veins: If you have a job that requires extended sitting or standing, regularly flex your leg muscles. You can do that inconspicuously simply by pressing the balls of your feet against the floor to flex the calf muscles. Short walks also will assist the veins in moving blood along, as can simply keeping the legs raised. Add a few Foot Circles, as described in the box "Wiggle as You Work," and you'll really be doing your veins a favor.

Wiggle as You Work

Even if you're desk-bound for most of the day, you can get the blood moving in your legs without ever leaving your chair. Veins like all the help they can get from muscles, so make a conscious effort to flex your leg muscles. Wiggle your toes frequently, and slowly raise and lower yourself on the balls of your feet. Once or twice a day try doing Foot Circles. With your legs extended, simply rotate your feet at the ankles—15 times in one direction, then 15 times in the other.

2. Fiber up. As prevalent as varicose veins are in the United States, they're virtually nonexistent in some less industrialized societies. The reason?

The constant exercise those people get is certainly a factor, but so is their diet. People in nonindustrial societies tend to eat lots of foods rich in fiber, and with fiber comes ease in moving the bowels. And yes, the easier life is for the bowels, the easier life is for the veins. Straining at stool can pass undue pressure on to the vascular system, aggravating weaknesses in vein walls or vein valves. So, tip number two for bettering

Pregnancy—Often the Start of Varicose Veins

Although varicose veins are far more prevalent in women (especially women who have had children) than in men, Howard C. Baron, M.D., a vascular surgeon, notes that pregnancy itself does *not* cause them. Instead, it's generally thought today that female *hormones,* especially those released during pregnancy, play a role in producing varicose veins in susceptible women. Frequently, inflamed veins may be the first sign of pregnancy, even before a missed menstrual period, but they often recede after delivery. Because the unsightly blue cords pop out before the veins come under increased pressure, this suggests the weight of the fetus may be less a factor than hormones.

Since the condition is aggravated by sitting or standing in one position for too long, exercises such as walking, swimming, cycling—anything that gets your legs moving—can work to keep blood from pooling in your legs.

Additionally, wearing elastic support stockings may help, as will elevating your legs several times throughout the day and staying within your doctor's weight-gain guidelines. Avoid constricting knee socks or too-tight boots, and never sit with your knees crossed.

your odds against varicose veins: Eat a diet rich in grains, fruits and vegetables. (You'll be doing your heart and waistline a favor, too.)

3. Wear support hose. Muscular contractions, as we've mentioned, can help move blood along from inside the leg, but properly fitting elastic support hose can lend similar assistance—from the outside. Says Victor Pellicano, M.D., an internist from Lewiston, New York, "Not only can support hosiery give comfort to those who already have varicose veins, it could delay the onset of the problem for many years in people who don't."

Commercially available support stockings are fine for most people, research has shown, but for people with great differences between the size of their calves and ankles, custom-fitted stockings often are needed. Tip number three for side-stepping varicosity: Get several good pairs of proper-fitting support stockings and use them.

So there you've got it: a three-pronged attack for preventing or alleviating varicose veins. The experts we talked to had a few more ideas for giving varicosity the runaround:

- Beware of restrictively tight clothing. On your blacklist should be tight-fitting calf-length boots, panty hose that are too snug at the groin and girdles and corsets too tight for comfort.
- Include citrus fruits in your diet. Citrus fruits (oranges, tangerines, grapefruit) contain vitaminlike substances called bioflavonoids, which research indicates may help maintain the strength of vein walls.
- Consider the toilet off-limits for reading. The shape of a hardwood or plastic seat can put undue pressure on the veins of the backs of the thighs, pressure that gets passed on to the veins of the lower legs. Keep those magazines and books on the coffee table or by the bed.

C H A P T E R
E L E V E N

Help for Troubled Knees

The human knee wasn't designed to withstand extreme punishment. This limitation caused the cloud that rained on the careers of Joe Namath, Gale Sayers, Mickey Mantle, Dick Butkus, Bubba Smith and hundreds of other athletes. Recent advances in microscopic surgery were all that saved Olympic gold medal gymnast Mary Lou Retton and marathoner Joan Benoit Samuelson from a similar fate.

Yet knee injuries don't savage just the famous. Thomas F. Griffin, Jr., M.D., a sports medicine expert from Douglas, Arizona, says that weekend athletes who suffer severe pain, hear a popping noise or tear or develop an unstable knee should seek immediate medical treatment. If your knee hurts when you bear weight or hurts for more than three days, see your doctor. For minor twists and sprains, Dr. Griffin suggests using a common pro football technique. Wrap the knee once with a long Ace bandage. Put ice over the first bandage layer, then finish by wrapping over the ice to secure it to the knee. Elevating the knee will also comfort it. Aspirin or ibuprofen can reduce inflammation and

How Sports Take Their Toll on the Knees

When it comes to joints, nothing takes a beating like the knees. But, of course, different activities are harder on the knees than others. This table shows the impact certain movements have on these joints. The weak-kneed would be wise to choose their sport accordingly.

Sport	Functions of the Knee							Total
	Bends	Straight-ens	Angles from Side to Side	Slides	Rolls	Rotates	Subject to External Force	
Ice hockey	4	4	5	5	5	5	5	33
Football	5	5	5	4	4	5	4	32
Basketball	5	5	5	4	4	4	3	30
Skiing	3	3	5	5	5	5	4	30
Soccer	5	5	5	4	4	4	3	30
Wrestling	4	4	4	4	4	4	4	28
Karate	4	4	3	3	2	4	4	24
Baseball	3	3	3	3	4	4	2	22
Running	5	5	3	2	2	2	2	21
Tennis	3	3	3	3	3	3	1	19
Swimming	3	3	3	2	2	2	1	16
Golf	2	2	3	2	2	3	1	15

SOURCE: Adapted from "Treatment of Injuries to Athletes: Special Problems of Runners and Joggers," by James D. Key (Dallas, Tex.: James D. Key Sports Medicine Clinics of America, Key Clinic Associated, 1978). Reprinted by permission of the author.

NOTE: 1 = little or no use; 2 = light use; 3 = medium use; 4 = strong use; 5 = very strong use.

deflate lingering pain. Dr. Griffin warns, however, that using drugs to dull the pain without seeing a doctor may result in further damage.

Keep Your Knee out of Trouble

To avoid knee trouble in the first place, Stanley G. Newell, M.D., a podiatrist from Seattle, Washington, offers these tips to prevent common knee injuries.

- Wear the proper shoes for individual sports and check for uneven wear.
- Make sure your shoes and supports fit properly.
- Increase your workout time or jogging mileage no more than 10 percent every other week.
- Shorten your strides when running downhill.
- If you change from a hard to soft or soft to hard playing or running surface, says Dr. Newell, divide your workouts between them the first few weeks to give your body time to adjust to the change.

Exercise for Knee Pain

Rocks and a sock can help prevent the knee pain that comes from the constant pounding of walking, running or jumping exercise, says Lisa Dobloug, a Washington, D.C., fitness consultant. Put two pounds of rocks, bolts, coins or sand in a sock and tie the end. Next, sit in a chair and drape the sock over your ankle, with the weight falling to both sides. Then raise and lower your calf, bending at the knee, about 20 times. Repeat with your other leg. Do the exercise once a day to help strengthen the knee muscle, ligaments and thigh muscle. "That will lessen the chance of injury," says Dobloug.

Simple Solutions for Foot and Heel Problems

With all the new information that's available about the care and maintenance of the human foot, there's really no reason for you to put up with foot pain any more. The same walking and jogging boom that introduced thousands of American soles to blisters and sore arches also mothered the invention of lots of useful foot-saving shoes, devices and exercises.

If you want to understand how to solve your foot problems, you should first understand what happens to your feet during locomotion.

Ideally, the outside edge of your heel is the first part of your foot to hit the ground when you run or walk. Take a step and you'll see right away that you land on your heel. After that, notice that your weight naturally shifts forward and across the arch to the ball of your foot. Then, as you're bringing your other leg around, all your weight balances for a split second on your big toe, which you push off with.

46

Why Feet Wear and Tear

Search the sole of your shoe. Those three spots—the outside of the heel, the ball of the foot and the big toe—should show the most wear and tear.

Active people tend to develop foot pain in two places. One of them is the heel. When you jog or run, your heels hit the ground with a force greater than your weight. The heel of a 150-pound jogger, it's been estimated, hits the ground with a force of 255 pounds, and the heel of a runner of the same weight hits the ground with a force of roughly 375 pounds—over and over and over.

Couple those statistics with the fact that the layer of fat globules that cushions our heels during youth becomes thinner and less resilient with age, and it's not surprising that heel pain strikes many an adult jogger.

The other area of trouble is the arch, and its problem has a fancy name: plantar fasciitis, or inflammation of the plantar fascia.

The plantar fascia is a tough band of fibrous tissue that crosses the sole, linking the heel bone to the ball of the foot. With every step we take, all our weight comes down on the fascia, pushing the arch down and in. In an exercise program of walking or running, excessive pronation (rolling in of the foot) causes more rapid pulling of the fascia from the bone.

In time, the fascia may stretch and become inflamed. It may even begin to tear away from the heel bone, causing the formation of a bony growth called a heel spur. Heel spurs themselves are seldom painful, but the increased pulling of the tissue away from the bone that often accompanies fasciitis is the most common source of foot pain among adults who exercise.

"A good percentage of the walking or jogging population has symptomless heel spurs to some extent," says Phillip Perlman, D.P.M., a Boulder, Colorado, podiatrist who specializes in runners' foot problems. "Jogging or running may speed up the separation process, thus producing painful symptoms."

How can a person tell if he has plantar fasciitis? "People can usually diagnose themselves," says Dr. Perlman, who often jogs with his patients to observe their form. "It's fasciitis if it feels like a stone bruise on the heel that won't go away, or if there's pain as soon as you roll out of bed in the morning."

What to Do

What should you do or not do about plantar fasciitis? Dr. Perlman advises against x-rays, for one thing. "X-rays are expensive, the body doesn't need the radiation exposure, and most of the time they aren't necessary," he says. Some podiatrists use injections of cortisone into the heel to stop the inflammation and pain, or perform surgery to separate the fascia from the heel bone. Dr. Perlman uses these options only when all else fails.

Ice is nice.   Ordinary ice may be the best treatment for fasciitis. One thing Dr. Perlman sometimes suggests to his patients is to put on two pairs of socks and then slip some ice between the two layers. Keep the ice there for about 20 minutes, he says, and repeat the process three to five times a day until the pain subsides.

Ice applied externally seems to help in any form. John Grady, D.P.M., of Chicago, tells his patients to fill a Styrofoam cup full of water, freeze it, then strip away the edge of the cup and massage the painful area with this cylindrical icicle as needed. Applying ice right after a workout seems to help many runners.

Foot baths.   In his book *Foot and Ankle Pain,* Rene Cailliet, M.D., of the University of California School of Medicine, says that gentle heat or cold both can help any sort of foot strain. Try cold first, then heat, he says, or alternate a cold foot bath with a warm one.

Arch and heel supports.   Many people try to prevent or cure their foot problems by shopping for an arch support or heel cushion that they can slip into their shoes. If this doesn't do the trick, then a professional orthotic may work better. An orthotic is an arch and heel support custom-made from a plaster cast of your foot. Orthotics can cost as much as $300, however, and most people look for something "off the rack" and less costly.

There are several kinds of inexpensive insoles designed to absorb the shock of walking and running. Scholl manufactures a green foam pad called Pro Comfort, as well as arch supports. Spenco makes a whole family of insoles and arch supports. Insoles made from a super-resilient material called Sorbothane are also popular, although some people say they're too heavy. These products are available in sporting-goods stores and stores that sell running shoes.

The right shoes.   Many foot-pain sufferers go searching for the ideal jogging shoe for their feet. Visit a runners' store and you'll find customers and salesmen in deep discussion about how much the customer runs or walks and what sort of support he needs. Since running shoes are expensive—up to $85 for one model—you might want to consult a sports-minded podiatrist before laying your money down.

There's also a new breed of shoes on the market that combines the handsome leather uppers of a street or casual shoe with the cushioning, light weight and rugged sole of a jogging shoe. The Rockport Company of Massachusetts offers a line of smart walking shoes called RocSports.

(continued on page 52)

Flexing the Feet

Certain exercises can help get you back on your feet if you've been laid up by foot pain. Here's one of them:

Slip off your shoes and sit with your feet dangling above the floor. With lots of energy, point your toes down, then in, then up and then out, so that you make circles in the air with your big toes. Simultaneously flex and extend your toes. Rene Cailliet, M.D., of the University of California School of Medicine, says these exercises strengthen your leg and foot muscles.

Here are a few exercises you can do while standing:

Place your feet apart and pointing in, as if you're a little pigeon-toed. Roll onto the outside of your feet several times and curl your toes tightly. Also, practice walking on your toes, slightly pigeon-toed. When you're walking to lunch or in the shopping mall, it also helps to purposely put some bounce into your stride.

Stretching your Achilles tendon can sometimes relieve heel pain. Stand a few feet away from a wall, facing it. Place one foot ahead of the other and then put both palms on the wall as if you were pushing a stalled car. Keep the knee of your rear leg straight, while keeping the heel of that leg on the floor. Bend your forward leg and raise that foot.

"Feel Great" Foot Massage

What could make your feet feel better than a foot massage? In fact, no matter what's hurting, "for every important organ or muscle area in the trunk and head there is a tiny area that corresponds to it on one or both feet," says George Downing, author of *The Massage Book.* A massage may really give an all-over, pain-relieving workout. What follows are Downing's directions for giving a great foot massage. He recommends little or no oil but considerable elbow grease—so press hard for best results.

1. Choose a comfortable place to work. If you're using a massage table, have your partner lie on his or her back. Otherwise, seat your partner in a chair with one foot propped on a cushioned stool. Start by holding the top of the foot with one hand. Make a fist with the other and massage the entire sole with your knuckles, using tiny circular movements from heel to toe. Don't forget the bottom of the heel.

2. Now grasp the foot with both hands, with your thumbs on the sole. Massage the sole again with your fingers and thumbs, pressing in the same circular motions. Go very slowly and carefully—you don't want to miss any pain-relieving spots. And don't forget to use a lot of pressure (about the same force you'd use to push a thumbtack into a piece of wood).

3. Change your grip and vigorously massage the top of the foot from toes to ankle, using the same thumb motions. As you approach the ankle and heel, massage with your

fingertips, but keep up the same circular pressure. Make
sure to massage both the top and sides of the ankle, then
end at the bottom of the heel.

4. Once you reach the bottom of the heel, lift the foot from
behind the ankle and use the fingertips and thumb of the
opposite hand to slowly massage the bottom edge of the
heel. Press firmly.

5. Now look at the top of the foot. See those long, thin
tendons running from the ankle to the toes? Run the tip
of your thumb down the valley between them, pressing
hard. When you reach the flap of skin between the
toes, give it a gentle squeeze before moving on to the
next valley.

6. Now point your thumbs away from the toes and bring
the heels of your hands together. Wrap your hands
around the foot and press firmly in both directions—
downward with the heels of your hands and upward with
your fingertips against the middle of the sole. Continue
steady pressure while slowly sliding the heels of your
hands apart. When they reach the outer edges of the
foot, start over. Do this three times.

7. Hold the foot steady and massage the toes. Grasp the
base of the big toe between your thumb and forefinger
and pull gently. Twist it gently from side to side as if you
were removing a cork from a bottle. Allow your fingers
to slide off the tip. Do each toe in turn.

8. Finally, cool down the foot by clasping it between your
palms, sandwich style. Hold it motionless for a few
moments before moving on to the other foot.

The Danner Shoe Company of Oregon makes a sturdy shoe called Danner Urban Lights. Podiatrists may recommend these shoes for salesmen, nurses, letter carriers and anybody else who stands or walks for a living.

How Professional Walkers Take Care of Their Feet

It's interesting to find out how people who walk for a living take care of their feet. Larry and Gale Forman, of San Diego, belong to that group. Seven years ago, the Formans started a walking association called Walkabout International, which organized walking tours of urban San Diego. Today, through Intimate Glimpses, a new enterprise that grew out of their original venture, the Formans organize and lead walking tours all over the world.

The Formans recently returned from a three-week tour of Switzerland. Within hours after their arrival home, they both received foot reflexology treatments. Reflexology is a specialized form of massage that involves kneading the soles of the feet. The Formans say that few things are as rejuvenating for the feet as a thorough reflexology treatment.

Blister prevention.   The Formans have also seen their share of blisters, and there's one product they recommend. It's called Second Skin and it's made by Spenco. Second Skin is a small piece of transparent film that's premoistened. It's designed to clean the wound, protect it from friction and hold moisture in. Moleskin, which is cloth with an adhesive backing, is a Scholl product that also seems to help blisters. Some people apply it in advance to prevent blisters wherever they usually get them. Ordinary white adhesive tape may also help.

Soft soaks.   A product called Johnson's Foot Soap comes highly recommended for the aches and pains of a walker's feet. Gary Yanker, a New York lawyer and author of *The Complete Book of Exercise Walking,* uses it regularly. On the market since 1870, Johnson's Foot Soap contains soap flakes, borax, iodine and bran. Mix one of the individual packages in two quarts of water, then soak your feet. It helps promote circulation and softens the tough outer layer of the foot. Yanker claims that it "works wonders."

Whirlpools. Whirlpool baths can also soothe aching feet. Many mailmen say that after beating the pavement all day, they sometimes head for the whirlpool at their local athletic club. A number of companies manufacture small household foot baths for between $30 and $80. Clairol makes one called Foot Fixer, while Pollenex makes one called Feet Relief.

Other Inside Tips

For added comfort—and good foot health—consider these words of advice:

Do walk on the grass. You can help your feet considerably by walking or jogging on grass instead of concrete. One podiatrist says that farmers, above all others, retain good foot structure throughout their lives because they spend so little time on hard pavement.

Lose excess weight. If you are overweight, losing weight might be the best way to take a load off your feet, podiatrists say.

Also, when your feet are hurting, arthritis, gout or diabetes could be the reason. Arthritis twists the bones out of shape, causing considerable pain when you walk. Gout, a condition caused by the deposit of uric acid crystals at the joints, may also be the source of the pain. Diabetes, which prevents good circulation in the extremities, is another possibility. All three of these conditions require a doctor's attention.

Ultimately, there's more at stake in the treatment of foot pain than just the comfort of your feet. The posture of our feet influences the bone structure of the whole body, and the health of the whole body often relies on the exercise we get while walking or running. Our feet, and how we care for them, can make all the difference.

Taming Tennis Elbow

The more you play, the more you pay. That's the way it is with tennis elbow. A survey done several years ago by orthopedic surgeon James D. Priest, M.D., showed that 45 percent of daily tennis players suffered from the condition, while only 7 percent of people playing two or three times a month had pain. People playing once or twice a week suffered at a rate of 26 percent.

"The overriding factor in the development of tennis elbow is frequency of play," the journal *The Physician and Sportsmedicine* commented on these findings.

The Physics of Tennis Elbow

So what actually causes tennis elbow?

A quick look at the physics of tennis should provide the answer. Before meeting the ball, the head of a racquet can reach speeds of 350 miles per hour. In the split second contact is made, however, racquet speed slows to about 150 miles per hour—quite a braking job, indeed, for the tendons of the elbow. Add a little faulty technique to this situation, or some rotation caused by an off-center hit, and you've really got an elbow under fire. Small tears can occur in tendons as the result of this abuse, and whammo: a case of tennis elbow.

R and R for Tennis Elbow

The first step in recovery is to give up the game for as long as your elbow is sore. While the tendons are healing, work on strengthening the forearm muscle with a five-pound dumbbell. Rest your arm on a table beside your chair, with the wrist extending over the edge. With the dumbbell in hand, slowly raise and lower the weight ten times. Rest one minute, then do ten more lifts. Repeat once more.

As the exercise becomes easier, you can increase the weight of the dumbbell. When your elbow stops hurting, you're ready for the courts again.

Three Gizmos to the Rescue

Naturally, you'll want to prevent tennis elbow from striking again. Certain products have responded with commendable intelligence to tennis elbow, and we report on three of them here. The CTE is a racquet uniquely designed to reduce both racquet twist and racquet vibration. The Power Mate is a combination wrist support and racquet stabilizer designed to prevent backhand errors that are known to encourage tennis elbow. And The Gripper helps protect the elbow by strengthening muscles of the hand and forearm.

The CTE Tennis Racquet.   Designed and produced by former commercial artist and tennis-elbow sufferer G. Chris Winkler, the primary mission of the CTE (Convex Torque Eliminator) is to reduce strain on the elbow by directing the force of ball contact toward the center of the racquet face in the case of off-center hits, thus minimizing the tendency of the racquet to twist. According to the manufacturer, the CTE performed this function very well in laboratory tests (scoring 35 percent higher in stability than all other 127 midsized racquets tested), and the racquet was praised for its "considerable torsion stability" by *Tennis* magazine. Players who've tried the CTE say that it does indeed have a massive "sweet spot," and that the racquet transmitted very little vibration—another suspected tennis-elbow antagonist. Four models of the CTE are available, with prices ranging from $120 to $280. For more information, contact the Chris Development Corporation, 122 South Sixth Avenue, West Bend, WI 53095 (800-336-9028 or 414-334-0311).

The Power Mate. The Power Mate attacks tennis elbow from a different angle—namely, the wrist. By helping to support a proper "right angle" grip, the Power Mate allows the hand and forearm muscles to rest from damaging movements as it corrects backhand technique. Designed by former sports medicine consultant to the Polish Olympic team Arthur Zaremba, M.D., the elastic support also claims to allow players a looser and less exhaustive grip. It's especially suited as a training device for beginners (no two-handed backhands, please). The Power Mate sells for $59.95 and is a product of the Institute for Sports Research, Inc., 4676 Admiralty Way, Suite 401D, Marina del Rey, CA 90292 (800-272-2334; in California, 800-833-9316).

The Gripper. Attacking tennis elbow from yet another angle is The Gripper—a squeezable exercise device that can reduce risks of tennis elbow by strengthening muscles responsible for preventing the condition in the first place. Experts agree that a weak grip and tennis elbow go hand in hand because a proper hold on the racquet handle is essential for a proper stroke. The Gripper is small enough to fit inconspicuously into a coat pocket. You simply squeeze it repetitively whenever you've got the chance, and in several weeks, its manufacturers say, you should have the forearm of Popeye. Priced at a very reasonable $3.99, The Gripper is available at most sporting-goods stores and is made by Triangle Health and Fitness Systems, Box 2000, Morrisville, NC 27560 (call 919-469-4111 for a retailer near you). The Gripper should not be used once tennis elbow has struck, however. "When tennis elbow is in the acute phase, you want to be resting it, not aggravating it," says Ray Hedenberg, a physical therapist with the Allentown Sports Medicine Clinic, Allentown, Pennsylvania.

Exercise for a Healthy Back

Can you get out of a car in one seamless motion? Work in your garden without wondering how you are going to straighten up at the end of the day? Make love with no fear that your body is going to kink up in some weird position that only an emergency medical team can undo?

You can if your spine is strong and flexible, able to bounce back from the stress of daily life. If it isn't that way with you, you can at least move in that direction by revitalizing the muscles, bone, cartilage and nerves that make up your spine. How? With a program of careful exercise, nutrition and lifestyle changes.

Some Background Information

Why are our backs so weak? Because we were a little hasty in getting up off all fours. About four million years ago, someone's brain said, "I think I could get more done if I didn't have to use my hands as feet." So that person stood up, and the rest of us followed. And our backs have been trying to catch up ever since.

Not that our backs are so archaic that we should be ashamed of them. The human spine is a wonderfully intricate structure. It's just that we are now asking it to function vertically when its basic design is still more suited for life on the horizontal. Indeed, virtually all common back problems are a result of downward pressure causing wear and tear on the bones of the spine (vertebrae) and the pads (disks) that separate them. Backache is a discouragingly "normal" development, says Hamilton Hall, M.D., author of *The Back Doctor.*

So what do we do with these backs of ours that can lock up on us at the drop of a hat?

We learn to live with them, Dr. Hall says. We learn to sit, stand, bend, lift, sleep, brush our teeth, bowl, have sex, work and give piggyback rides with them. Because, in time, most back problems will cure themselves. Studies show, in fact, that backache is more of a middle-age problem than an old-age problem. By the time we turn 60 or so, our backs usually have made do with the imperfections that can cripple us in our thirties.

With that in mind, surgery, Dr. Hall says, should be avoided at all costs. "Fewer than 5 percent of all people with back pain are likely to benefit from surgery," he reports. "At least 19 out of 20, including serious cases, are better off with some combination of physiotherapy, medication, exercise and what we refer to as proper ADL—activities of daily living."

We'll explain those activities shortly. But first we've got to consider what kind of back problem you might have. Dr. Hall says all common backaches are due to:

- A worn facet joint (which he calls Type One);
- A protruding disk (Type Two);
- A pinched nerve (Type Three); or, unfortunately,
- A combination of two, or even all three, of these factors.

The following descriptions may help you get an idea of what may be causing your discomfort.

Type One—a worn facet joint.   This type of problem hurts most "when you arch your back, as you would when you lean back to look up at the ceiling," Dr. Hall says. The pain you feel is mainly at the top of your buttocks, and you find that bending slightly forward tends to relieve it. "Your trouble begins with a minor incident of routine exertion, such as picking up a garden hoe or retrieving a golf ball," according to Dr. Hall, and it usually subsides, if you rest it, within 4 to 14 days. If your problem is Type One, you probably experience such attacks two or three times a year.

Type Two—a protruding disk. This pain shares many of the symptoms of Type One, but it also has these distinguishing differences, Dr. Hall says: "A Type Two attack may begin with the same sort of incident as Type One, but the onset of pain is likely to be less sharp and immediate; more often it will build up slowly, over a couple of days, from mild discomfort to severe pain. The pain will recede noticeably in a week or two, but, unlike Type One pain, it won't disappear. Instead, it will linger on as a nagging backache or, in some cases, as an intense and constant pain." Unlike Type One, though, Type Two isn't aggravated more when you bend back; it's bending forward that intensifies the pain. "Like Type One, Type Two pain is felt mainly in the back, although it may radiate into the buttocks and legs," Dr. Hall explains, "just as Type One does."

Type Three—a pinched nerve. You might think of this as Type Two Plus, Dr. Hall says, because it involves a disk that has protruded to the point of pressing on a nerve. Hence, it has many of the symptoms of Type Two pain but also some of its own: pain can extend not just into the thighs but also lower, sometimes even to the feet and toes. Type Three pain usually comes on over a day or two, builds, and then stays for weeks. It is made distinctly worse by bending forward, and it is potentially the most serious of the three types because prolonged pressure can damage nerve function. It is also the least common, however, and it is responsible for only about 10 percent of all back woes.

What causes these three types of back pain?

In the case of Type One pain, it's usually a disk that has flattened to the point of allowing the bones of a facet joint to rub against one another. Disks can flatten because of a gradual drying-out process (a natural consequence of aging), and that process can be hastened by a life of hard physical labor and heavy lifting. It can also be aggravated by bad posture, pregnancy or a potbelly, because anything that causes you to arch your back causes facet joints (located at the back of the spine) to press together.

Type Two back pain is the result of a disk doing more bulging than collapsing, because disks are not "dead" tissue. They contain nerve fibers, and they hurt when they get pushed out of shape.

Type Three back pain is the result of a disk bulging to the point of pressing on a spinal nerve—one of the few cases in which surgery may be required for repair.

How to Help Your Back Feel Stronger

Maybe now you can see why bed rest is so often recommended as the first order of business following a back attack. By lying down, you relieve pressure on disks, which in turn relieves pressure on spinal nerves, which should in turn erase the reason for the muscles of your back going into painful—but protective—spasm. Muscle spasms are your body's way of encouraging the very immobilization you need in order to heal. And not until those spasms relax is it time to think about doing some corrective exercises —exercises, as strange as it may sound, that concentrate not on the back but on the stomach.

Why the stomach?

Because strong stomach muscles can provide a weak back with the additional support it needs. When stomach muscles are weak, greater pressure gets passed on to the disks, which are too important to strain.

Abdominal exercises, however, are not the entire answer to getting along with a bad back. As we mentioned earlier, there are those all-important activities of daily living—ADLs, as Dr. Hall calls them. The idea is to make life as easy on your back as possible in as many situations as possible.

How to sleep. If you sleep on your back, roll a couple of pillows into a bolster to raise up your knees. Or, if you prefer sleeping on your stomach, "try sleeping with a pillow under the front of your pelvis to reduce the sag in your lower back," Dr. Hall says. Side sleepers should curl into a ball and place a pillow between their knees. The purpose of all these positions is to reduce pressure on spinal disks.

How to stand. Assume the "S" stance. The trick to standing, and walking, is to find a posture that feels comfortable but offers your back maximum support. "We want to maintain the gentle 'S' curve of the spine," says Terry Nordstrom, director of the department of physical and occupational therapy and originator of the Back School of Stanford University. For some, in the case of swayback, it helps to pull in the stomach and tuck under the buttocks. This tilts the pelvis toward the back and provides crucial support for the lower spine. Keep your knees slightly flexed, too.

"Never stand flat-footed if you can put one foot up on a stool or a low shelf—the posture drinkers assume at a stand-up bar. That prevents the knees from locking and takes pressure off the lower back. Saloonkeepers discovered the comfort of this position long before doctors developed the theory behind it," Dr. Hall says.

How to sit.   The first rule of thumb is not to sit for very long. Sitting can create a greater load on spinal disks than standing. You can reduce that load by making sure to support yourself with your elbows if you must lean forward to work at your desk. In other, more recreational sitting situations, try to keep your feet raised—on either a step stool or a stack of books—and place a small pillow between the back of your chair and the area just above your buttocks.

How to lift.   Lift with your back as straight as possible. Squat, in other words, but don't bend over. The more work you can pass on to the legs, the better. "The most hazardous lifts are the ones for which you are unprepared," Dr. Hall says. And the most difficult, even when you are prepared, are the ones where you must hoist something over a barrier at arm's length—for example, a 40-pound nephew out of a high-sided crib. Make it a habit to think before you attempt a lift. If even the thought of it hurts, chances are that it will.

One place to learn how to lift things without lowering your spirits is a book by a physics professor at Tufts University in Massachusetts. Physics is, among other things, the study of the movement of bodies in space, and so there is no better person to tell you how to lift the miscellaneous weights of your life than a physics teacher. Jack R. Tessman, Ph.D., in his practical and very likable volume *My Back Doesn't Hurt Anymore,* strips the he-man show-off and the "Don't worry; I can do it myself" from most lifting jobs and treats them like the mechanical problems he teaches his students. What's the best, most efficient way to get this job done? he asks in each case.

In brief, Dr. Tessman's advice is that you shouldn't bend forward to pick up anything unless there's something there to support your weight.

The physics behind this advice is simple and straightforward. Imagine that you and a friend want to ride on a seesaw at the neighborhood playground. Your friend weighs 100 pounds and sits down five feet away from the pivot point at the center of the plank. You sit down on the other side of the plank but only a foot away from the pivot point. To balance your friend, you would have to weigh 500 pounds.

Now imagine your body as a seesaw. Your arms, reaching down and forward, are like your friend's half of the plank. Your hips are like the pivot point. Now your lower back muscles strain to lift that load. But since they are close to your hips, they have no leverage. It has been estimated that, in an activity such as shoveling, the back muscles must pull with a force 15 times the weight of the object lifted.

The solution to this problem is simply to lift and carry things beside or behind you, making the load work with your back muscles instead of against them.

How to have sex.   There are a number of pain-free techniques: face-to-face, with both partners on their sides; or face-to-back, in what is sometimes called the "spoon" position, with the woman nestled against the man's lap. There are, of course, many other possible positions, and the key to avoiding strain "is to make sure you do not arch your back or your neck" in all of them, says Dr. Hall.

A Day's Worth of Lifting

Imagine, for a moment, a normal day:

The alarm clock is ringing; it's 6:00 A.M. Getting out of bed is your back's first test of the day. Push yourself up and forward with your hands, and swing your feet around.

Next stop is the bathroom. When shaving or washing your face, take a load off your back by flexing at the knees or supporting your weight with a free hand. Then, while you're dressing, bring your foot up instead of bending forward to slip on socks or stockings.

Outside, on the welcome mat, lies the morning newspaper. Instead of bending over, flex at the knees and keep your back as straight as possible.

At breakfast, even little exertions such as reaching into the refrigerator for a gallon jug of milk or reaching across the table for a platter of eggs could aggravate an existing back problem. Later, before you go out for the day, you might want to give your child or grandchild a bear hug. Avoid reaching over a crib railing or a safety gate to pick him up. Instead, lower the railing or open the gate and flex your knees rather than bending over.

Assuming that you have been to work and are now ready to come home (there's no room here to cover the multitude of hazards on the job), you might stop to buy groceries. Supermarkets can pose a real dilemma for someone with a bad back. Heavy-duty paper bags are loaded too heavily, and deep-well shopping carts create awkward lifting situations.

Instead of one big sack, try carrying two smaller ones, one under each arm. If you can, use the new carts with waist-level bottoms. When loading bags into the car, don't put them on the floor. Put them on a seat or on the rear deck if you have a station wagon.

In spring and summer, you may want to knock around the garden after work. If you're spading compost or soil, keep the payload end of the spade at your side or behind you. Dr. Tessman even suggests digging behind you, as if you were paddling a canoe. If you're putting in seeds, kneel rather than lean over and, if you kneel, use your forearm to prop up your weight.

Changing tires is another chore that can be a disaster for your back. To avoid the crunch, squat or sit on a stool when you pull off the tire and wheel. When loosening the lug nuts, always push down with the wrench.

Back inside the house, it might be time to open a window that's hard to budge. If you face the window and pull up on the handles or grips, your back will think you're trying to lift the house. Instinct may tell you to do it that way, but it's far better to put your back to the window and raise it behind you.

The same principle applies to carrying a trunk, a sofa or an air conditioner: Hold the end that you're carrying behind you.

The day is almost done. You might want to give your child or grandchild a ride on your shoulders before he or she gets swaddled up and sent to bed. If you let the child use a sofa or chair to climb on your shoulders, you won't hurt your back. (For women who want to take infants with them during the day, what's best for their back is to carry the child on the back in a knapsacklike carrier.)

Your last chore of the evening involves that hallowed ritual: taking out the trash. If you try to carry a loaded trash can in front of you, by the handles, your back may never forgive you. Get your teenage son to take it down to the curb or drag the can behind you or best of all, put the can on a cart with wheels.

The Right and Wrong Exercises

Along with giving advice, Dr. Tessman also punctures a few myths about the back. Strong arm and back muscles, he says, can't protect your disks. On the contrary, someone with strong back muscles is more likely to pick up a load that's too heavy for the disks.

Certain traditional exercises are also taboo. Dr. Tessman says that bending over to touch your toes and doing Sit-Ups place unnecessary strain on the disks. He prefers Deep Knee Bends for strengthening the thigh muscles and deep breathing exercises for developing the abdominal muscles.

Here are six exercises recommended by back-care experts for people with backaches due to muscular problems. Before starting any exercise program, be sure to check with your doctor, especially if you are experiencing any pain. Keep in mind that each back problem is different—these exercises will relieve many people's back problems, but not everyone's. If you're not satisfied with the results, you may want to check with a back-care expert, who can individualize exercises to treat your problem.

Exercises for your back accomplish two goals. First, they strengthen muscles made weak through years of inactivity and improper posture. The key muscles you need to strengthen are the front and side abdominals. These support your spine and take a lot of weight off your back muscles. The Pelvic Tilt and the Modified Sit-Up work toward this goal.

Second, back-pain sufferers need exercises to stretch tensed-up, tightened muscles, especially those in the back, hips and legs. The more flexible the muscles in these areas are, the less vulnerable you are to back problems. The Cobra, Cat Back, Chair Bend and Knee-to-Chest Stretch all work on increasing flexibility.

Pelvic Tilt. This is a technique invented by Robert Lowe, M.D., an orthopedic surgeon and founder of the Low Back School at Cabell Huntington Hospital in West Virginia. Dr. Lowe explains that most of the forward and back bending of the spine takes place in the joint between the fifth (last) lumbar vertebra and the sacrum, which is the heavy bone forming the back of the pelvis. (It is really five vertebrae fused into one.) The sacrum is rather rigid compared to the fifth lumbar vertebra, and bending, lifting and even prolonged sitting put stress on the muscles, ligaments and disk that make up that joint. Ideally, strong stomach and buttock muscles will keep this part of the spine correctly aligned, but over time poor posture, sedentary habits and overweight can combine to accentuate the natural lumbar curve, producing a swaybacked, potbellied appearance. The stress from such a weakened condition falls most heavily on the joint between the fifth lumbar vertebra and the sacrum, and the Pelvic Tilt is an exercise designed to help reverse the curve temporarily, easing pressure on the disks and strengthening the supporting muscles. It is incredibly effective, considering its simplicity.

While lying on your back, bend your knees and place your feet flat on the floor near your buttocks. Raise your pelvis and "tuck" it under, concentrating on pushing your lower back gently to the floor. Your shoulders, legs, neck and upper back should be relaxed. As you gently push your lower back to the floor, three things begin to happen: your pelvis rotates forward (reversing the curve of your lower back), your buttock muscles tighten and your stomach muscles are exercised. If it's easy, you're in pretty good shape and will be able to keep your back near to or on the floor without straining. If you find it difficult, your back needs work. For some people, the Pelvic Tilt becomes an automatic part of their posture with little training. For others, it requires a great deal of effort.

Inside your back, the benefits from this simple exercise are great: the pressure on the rear part of the lumbar disks is eased, the stretched muscles and ligaments are relaxed and the supportive muscles of the stomach, buttocks and pelvis are toned and exercised.

You can and should also perform the Pelvic Tilt while standing.

(continued on page 68)

How to Avoid Runner's Backache

Most runners experience blisters or a sore knee, at least occasionally. But if your training gives you a pain in the back, it may be because of the way you run. To minimize stress on your spine, you should use your trunk and abdominal muscles as you run to keep the spine in a balanced, comfortable, neutral position. If you are flat-footed or knock-kneed or have one leg significantly shorter than the other, your particular style of pavement pounding may put considerable stress on vulnerable disks and spinal joints.

Where you run could also be part of the problem. Striding over uneven terrain or up and down hills can force an unprotected spine into uncomfortable positions. You may find relief by rerouting your runs over flatter ground or adjusting your style so that your shoes, ankles, knees and hips absorb more of the jolt of hitting the ground.

Muscle Power

Adjusting how and where you run can help lighten the load on your spine. But the real secret of a healthy lower back is having strong abdominal, back, hip and thigh muscles. And while running can help tone those muscles, they'll benefit even more from individual attention. Partial or isometric Sit-Ups go far to strengthen abdominal muscles. (Avoid full Sit-Ups; they put excessive stress on your spine.) If you have access to a weight machine, you can concentrate on several different exercises that will get these muscle groups in shape. Swimming is another good bet.

Once you've toned up your muscles, you'll find it easier to improve your body mechanics. By tightening your abdominal musculature, flexing your knees slightly and using your hip muscles and the rotational capabilities of your hips you can learn to hold your spine in a neutral balanced position while accomplishing virtually any task—including your daily run.

A New Way to Run

If your back pain is a recurring ailment, you may need to do something that sounds extreme and undesirable: Change your running style. You've probably been running in the same fashion for several years, and switching to a style that's kinder to your back is bound to slow you down, at least in the beginning. But if altering how you run is the only way for you to continue to run at all, the change is probably worth the effort.

You won't be able to relearn your running style overnight. And running is really the final step in a process that starts with you literally flat on your back.

Begin by lying on your back with your knees bent and your feet flat on the floor. Flatten your lower back against the floor and tighten your abdominal muscles. Press or pound against your stomach with a fist so that you can feel your tightened muscles. If you raise your shoulders and shoulder blades off the floor, you'll pull the abdominals even tighter.

Get used to what this feels like. Try to talk, sing or count with your muscles taut. Practice this technique until you're able to keep your shoulder blades off the floor for three minutes. That simple-sounding goal may take you several weeks to achieve.

Once you've made yourself a three-minute man or woman, you'll be ready for the second step. Stand with your back flat against a wall and your knees slightly bent. Tighten your abdominals as you did on the floor, and again practice breathing and talking while your muscles are tight. Next, push yourself away from the wall and stand up unsupported, but with your abdominals still tight and your knees flexed. Take a few steps without loosening your abdominal grip. When you get tired, lean against the wall again with your back flat and your knees flexed. Relax, then walk again.

With practice, you'll be able to take more and more steps with your abdominal muscles in their tightened, spine-protecting position. Concentrate on keeping your spine flat as you move.

(continued)

How to Avoid Runner's Backache—
Continued

Walk faster and faster and farther and farther. If your back pain returns, you haven't yet found the kind of balanced, neutral position that makes things easy on your spine. Keep experimenting. Depending on your underlying problem, you may need a little more swayback or slump in your back. If you can't find any position that feels comfortable, you may have to see a specialist for examination and diagnosis.

Once you can walk for a mile or two with your abdominal muscles tightened, start carrying hand weights. Walk rapidly, with your muscles taut. If you can do that without back pain, you're ready to run.

At first, jog slowly in a semicrouched position with your knees bent slightly. This should be nothing more than a quick-paced walk. Make sure your abdominals are tight and that your feet aren't slapping the ground. Try to run *softly.* You'll probably find this strenuous and somewhat awkward.

When you've mastered this new way of running, you can begin to straighten out of your crouch and move more normally. Make certain, though, to run softly, with your abdominals always tight. You should be able to do this without pain. If your back does hurt, you'll have to return to an earlier step in the sequence. Look for a position in which you're able to keep your spine comfortably stable.

Stand with your lower back against a wall and your feet six inches from it. Keep your lower back tight against the wall with your heels, buttocks and shoulders also touching it. Again, your neck, shoulders and legs are relaxed, and your stomach and buttock muscles are taut. In time, you should be able to assume the Pelvic Tilt posture without a supporting wall.

Can such a simple exercise really help? If faithfully practiced, the answer is yes. The benefits of the Pelvic Tilt have been documented by precise measurements of the pressure inside the spine. When you sit upright, 300 pounds of pressure per square inch is bearing on your lumbar disks (if you are of average weight); when you are standing, the pressure is 200 pounds; and when you are lying flat on your back, 100 pounds is brought to bear on the area. But lying in the Pelvic Tilt position reduces the force to 60 pounds per square inch!

Modified Sit-Up. Lie on your back with your knees bent. Don't anchor your feet. Put your hands on your thighs, or just stretch your arms out straight. Raise yourself up, while exhaling, until your fingertips reach your knees (about half of a regular Sit-Up). Hold for five seconds. Lower yourself back to the floor. Do just a few at first, and work up to 15 repetitions.

Cobra. Lie on your stomach with your hands in position as if you were about to do a Push-Up. Push your upper body off the floor until your arms are straight. Keep your hips on the floor and hold for about 15 seconds.

Cat Back. Get down on your hands and knees and arch your back upward, touching your chin to your chest. Breathe out deeply. Now return to the flat position and gently arch your back downward, like a suspension bridge. Hold and breathe deeply. Hold each position for about five seconds. Repeat six to eight times.

Chair Bend. Sit on a chair with your knees apart and your forearms on your thighs. Drop and sag at the shoulders and bend at the waist, breathing out as you bend. Drop your hands, lower your head between your knees and let your hands touch the floor. Hold for five seconds. Come up slowly by uncurling. Repeat six times.

Knee-to-Chest Stretch. Lie on your back with your knees bent. Bring your left knee up to touch your chest, hold for about 15 seconds, then lower your leg back to your original position. Be sure to stretch both legs, and repeat at least three times.

Now, the Upper Berth

So we've seen the good, the bad and the achy in troublesome backs, and we're done, right? Wrong! We're only half done, in fact. Up until now we've talked mainly about muscular and skeletal distortions of the spinal column and those of just the lower back to boot. We must still talk about pain in the upper back and, of course, in the neck. Fortunately, much of that task is accomplished by merely saying, "Ditto." Most of the things that go wrong with the lower back can also go wrong with the upper back, and they're avoided and treated in the same way. One problem that's very common in the upper reaches of the spine (and not so common down below) is the tightness and pain that's caused by the stress, miscellaneous distress and fatigue of getting through even normal days. *That* we must talk about.

Pain in the upper back and shoulders afflicts almost as many people as low back pain, which is the most common back problem. As in so many other illnesses, our backs are the victims of the city life, the sitting-down way of life.

The way we live and work in our modern society puts too much of the wrong kind of stress on this part of the body. For most of our daily activities, we sit over a desk, bench, typewriter, sewing machine or steering wheel. While washing dishes, cooking, typing or driving, our arms are always in pretty much the same position, straight out in front of us. If we lived a more rural life, our daily chores would guarantee plenty of twisting and very little sitting in the same tensed position.

Poor posture of this type causes a gradual buildup of tension, which affects the many nerve pathways in this area that control the hands, arms, head, heart, lungs and upper abdomen. Hour after hour of this tension builds up to a point where the tightness follows us to bed. We wake up with numb arms, a painful back or a headache.

Are You Your Back's Worst Enemy?

Keep in mind that many of our daily routines are potential trouble-makers and that taking early steps to strengthen the upper back will prevent attacks of severe stiffness and pain in the future.

Ask yourself if your working and playing hours put a lot of strain on this area. If you spend hours sitting in a stooped position over a desk or bench or steering wheel, you're probably giving little or no motion to the upper spine—motion it needs to stay healthy and loose. Of course, we occasionally have the natural protective reaction to this poor posture in the form of restlessness or the desire to get up and stretch.

Giving in to that urge is sometimes all that's needed. But it's important to do it frequently enough to make sure the effects of poor posture don't climb into bed with you. If you don't get rid of them by bedtime, you may wake up with aching shoulders and a stiff, painful upper back.

There is nothing as helpful as regularly moving these tense areas, which is what nature tries to tell us with the "restlessness reflex." Truck drivers, for instance, can make a habit of turning their head to look over their shoulder frequently, and stop every two hours for a good five-minute stretch and a short walk. And this advice is good for anyone who must be at the wheel for long periods at a time. Modern cars are made so low that the seats are more conducive to sleeping than to paying attention to the road. To overcome that, the driver has to thrust his or her head forward and concentrate, with little or no motion given to the upper back. This builds up tension. How often have you heard people say that they must rest up after a long driving trip? You won't need that rest at the end of your trip if you follow these suggestions for stretching and relaxing during the trip.

Most likely, however, it's really posture that is giving your upper back a bad time. Check your posture for round shoulders or a stooped position. Does one shoulder tilt downward or more forward than the other? Do your head and neck assume an erect, straight position? Do you spend much of your time at a bench or desk? If so, your upper back pain is probably the result of poor posture. And the sooner you establish a routine that will prevent back and shoulder problems, the better your health will be. (See the next chapter for more information on posture.)

Sitting Pretty, Standing Tall: A Guide to Better Posture

You may wonder why posture warrants a chapter in a book on trouble spots. The fact is that posture can exaggerate a bulging tummy, a sunken chest or a sagging bosom. Good posture, on the other hand, evens out a plump midsection, lifts your chest and alters your overall appearance for the better.

What is normally referred to as posture is merely the relationship of various parts of the body to each other. Though most people think posture is only the way we stand, it really is the way we carry ourselves at all times, whether standing, sitting or lying down.

Is Poor Posture Ruining Your Appearance?

According to Benjamin S. Golub, M.D., chief of the back service at the Hospital for Joint Diseases and Medical Center in New York, a strong, straight posture is no luxury. "You need good posture for all activities, including standing, sitting and bending." So find a full-length mirror and see what good posture looks like on you.

Stand erect, keeping your body firm, yet flexible.

Relax.

Look straight ahead and distribute your weight evenly on the ball of each foot, not the toes or heel. You should be able to raise your heels without leaning forward.

Slightly tilt your lower pelvis forward and upward. Imagine that you're holding a coin between your buttocks and you'll feel them tightening (don't bend your knees). As you shift into position, your buttocks should tuck in and the small of your back—the lumbar curve—should flatten into a slight arc.

"And flattening the lumbar curve," says Dr. Golub, "is the name of the game."

Hold your chest high. As you raise your chest, your shoulders naturally roll back and your stomach pulls in. (A slumping chest or sagging abdomen restricts your ability to breathe efficiently and comfortably.) But don't arch your back and suck in your stomach; this only develops the tense posture of a soldier at attention. "The military style of posture is too rigid," warns Dr. Golub. "Don't be a martinet."

A Checklist for a Straighter, Younger-Looking Stance

Your goal is good vertical alignment. That is, you should be able to drop an imaginary plumb line from just behind your ear through your shoulder and your sacrum (the last bone of the spine and part of the pelvis), behind your hip and your knee, and through your ankle.

Keep your chin level, straightening your neck into a vertical position.   For practice, you can look in a mirror, grasp a tuft of hair from the center of your head and pull up gently, aligning your chin parallel to the floor. Such neck and head adjustments should make you look taller and your neck look longer.

Hold your chest high.   Relax your shoulders and allow your arms to hang easily at your sides. As you do, your shoulders will automatically pull back where they should be and your bust will appear larger or more prominent. If you're executing the maneuver properly in a standing position, your palms will rotate inward to face your thighs.

Stand tall. This trick can make you look inches thinner because a shortened stomach muscle, caused by slumping, makes you appear paunchy. It's the aesthetic complement—and to some extent the natural result—of raising your chest.

Stand with your feet parallel. Don't point your toes outward, and distribute your weight evenly between the front and back of your feet. If you're standing properly, you shouldn't be able to see your heels when you look at your feet in a mirror. The stance enables you to maintain the erect and graceful posture you want. In the toes-outward position your knees lock and your lower pelvis is tilted backward—the prelude to a slumped posture.

Although it sounds like quite a goal—connecting all those bones—there are only four maneuvers to remember. Stand erect. Tilt your pelvis. Raise your chest. Tuck in your rear end. Everything else takes care of itself and falls naturally into place.

Don't be discouraged if you find yourself twisting like a go-go dancer in front of the mirror while trying to align your body. Chances are your body is accustomed to being "out of line," and at first good posture may seem uncomfortable or unnatural, creating tension in your lower back. But with time—and practice—you will be at ease.

Good posture, then, is a skill, just like playing a musical instrument or riding a bicycle. And, like other skills, it will improve steadily with practice. No matter how bad things look in the mirror, a little determination will go a long way to straighten out your reflection. Once you make up your mind to put in the effort, in fact, you may be surprised at how easy it is to improve your posture.

The Secrets of Better Posture

According to Raymond Harris, M.D., author of *Guide to Fitness after 50,* there are three basic parts to the process.

First, he says, be aware of your posture. Monitor your posture in mirrors and store windows instead of combing your hair or straightening your clothes.

"The idea," explains Dr. Harris, "is to mobilize your thought processes. The best way I know to do this is to walk as though you were wearing a crown."

Second, consciously place yourself in the proper positions. Dr. Harris suggests that you practice lying flat on the floor or on a slantboard (a piece of wood built on a slant so that you can rest with your feet higher than your head) or on a wide, strong ironing board with the small end propped up about six to ten inches. In this position your spine will straighten and your back will flatten. Muscles are relaxed and at ease. Small pillows can be placed behind your neck and knees to ease any strain on the spine.

The final component of the good posture process is stretching, massaging and exercising your muscles.

"Gentle massage is especially helpful for those over 50," says Dr. Harris. For some, he also recommends hanging from a chinning bar: "It stretches muscles gently and gets them working properly. It brings the back into proper alignment and relieves pressure on the nerves and disks."

Even rolling around on a padded or carpeted floor is beneficial. Dr.

Pregnancy and Posture

Oh, those pregnancy backaches! Poor posture, perhaps? Gail Sforza Brewer, childbirth educator and author, says, "Yes, when you're pregnant, your whole body changes. For physiological reasons, your back is more prone to strain. A lot of things happen inside the body, which allow everything to sort of loosen and soften to accommodate necessary stretching during childbirth. And the weight of the enlarged uterus, due to the relaxing of the abdominal muscles, can pull the spine into a curve. Sitting and standing erect will prevent this. It also can improve the circulation."

Brewer suggests using a foam wedge angled at 45 degrees under your back while sleeping as a posture aid. "You will be able to breathe much better and your lower back will be supported," she explains.

Harris claims it restores joint mobility by improving muscle tone and helps the muscles hold the body in proper posture.

When you think about posture, don't overlook the importance of proper breathing, he adds. Diaphragmatic, or belly, breathing is the basis for really good health.

Take a moment and try it.

Place your hand between your navel and ribs and take a deep breath. Your hand goes out as your diaphragm drops. Exhale, and your hand goes inward as the diaphragm rises. Again, practice makes perfect.

Stretching Is Good for Your Posture

Some of these exercises can even be done at your desk.

Sit Stretch I.   Sit with your back straight against a chair and put your feet flat on the floor. Fold your arms across the top of your head. Grasp your elbows with your fingers and squeeze for five seconds. Relax and repeat.

Sit Stretch II.   Sit with your back against a chair. Put your arms behind the chair, clasp your forearms and pull your shoulders back. Relax and repeat.

Knee Hold.   Sit with your back straight against a chair and your feet flat on the floor. Lift one knee and grasp it with your hands. Pull your knee toward your chest as far as you can without straining. Relax and repeat with the other leg.

Shoulder Stretch.   Stand as straight as possible and clasp your hands behind your head. Pull your elbows up and back as far as possible and hold for three seconds. Relax and repeat.

Leg Out.   Stand erect with your hands clasped behind your head. Get up on your toes and then swing one leg forward, keeping it straight and your toes pointed down. Return to the starting position and repeat with your other leg.

Bend.   Stand straight with your feet together and clasp your hands behind your back, keeping your arms extended. Then bend over at the waist and raise your clasped hands as high as you can above your shoulders. Return to the starting position and repeat.

Sculpting a New You

Sculpt the human body? Carve a new, firmer, trimmer you? It sounds too good to be true, but according to Ralph Carnes, Ph.D., former dean of the College of Arts and Sciences at Roosevelt University in Chicago, it's possible. The secret to body sculpting is working out with weights.

Dr. Carnes, coauthor of *Bodysculpture: Weight Training for Women,* claims that weight training is not just for men who want monumental muscles. It's for men *and* women who want well-toned muscles packed in a shape to be proud of. "You can zero in on your body's trouble spots," he says, "and sculpt a shapelier leg or firm a flabby arm with exercises aimed at those areas."

Weight training, like any exercise, burns calories, and that can mean an overall loss of extra fat. But just as important, lifting weights can enhance muscles in specific areas of the body, giving those areas a firmer and sleeker look. Thus, without losing an ounce, says Dr. Carnes, you can appear to have shaved off pounds.

But is there a danger that weight training will make women look like female versions of Arnold Schwarzenegger? Not really, says Ronald Mackenzie, M.D., medical director of the National Athletic Health Institute in Inglewood, California. "Women normally don't have the amount of male hormones it takes to build bulging muscles," he says. And they have an extra layer of fat that will mute muscle definition and guarantee soft curves, not rugged mountains.

Body-Building Goals for the "Average Person"

Spot *reducing* may not work, but spot *building* does.

Just how far you can take the concept of self-sculpting your body is another question. There is little question that muscle enhancement occurs most rapidly in males between the ages of about 15 and 25, thanks to the peak levels of male hormones during those years. In older men, muscle enlargement proceeds somewhat more slowly. By age 50, a man who has not previously done resistance training has no chance of ever looking like Hercules, although with any luck, he might wind up looking like Hercules' father.

What about women? It used to be said that women, regardless of age, could not develop large, rippling muscles because the right hormones weren't there. Now that many women have taken up body building as a hobby, that statement can no longer be made so glibly. Women *can* have large, well-developed muscles, although for sheer massiveness they aren't in the same league as men's muscles.

Body sculpting, or body building, as it is more commonly known, involves different exercises—in fact, a whole different philosophy— than exercising for pure brute strength alone. Basically, the person seeking great strength as his or her major goal will work out with relatively heavy weights (once properly warmed up, of course) and perform only a few repetitions at a time, typically three to six. And, again generally speaking, the exercises performed will concentrate on the muscles of the torso, back, chest and hips, with a secondary emphasis on the major muscle groups of the arms and legs.

Body builders take a different route. They usually use lighter weights but do more repetitions, typically between 8 and 15, but sometimes as many as 25. And they generally perform a much greater variety of exercises to make sure that every muscle in the body is thoroughly exercised.

Most body builders have such elaborate routines that they cannot complete an entire workout in one day. One day they may do ten different exercises for the upper body, repeating each exercise or "set" from three to six times. On the next day, they may work the muscles of the legs, abdomen or back. That approach not only enables the body builder to work every muscle but permits an important day of recuperation for each muscle, too. (Recuperation days are important to every resistance trainer, because stressful exercise actually produces minor damage to muscles even as it encourages their growth.)

The high number of repetitions performed by body builders is what leads to the striking increase in size and visibility, or what's called definition. After performing several sets of exercises, the body builder's muscles become engorged with blood and feel hot and stiff—"pumped," as they say in gyms. But still more exercise sets for the same muscles may follow, even though the muscles now have become so fatigued that they can handle only little more than half the weight they were working out with 20 minutes before. Yet, this is exactly the part of the workout that body builders feel does them the most good and produces the most dramatic results.

For most of us, though, three or perhaps four sets of any given exercise are all we need to stimulate impressive muscle growth.

How Body Building Works

If you're wondering just what weight training entails, here's a quick definition. Weight training is an exercise program that involves working the muscles against gradually increasing degrees of resistance. It differs from exercises such as jogging and racquetball—which obviously give your muscles a workout—by employing the "overload principle." That is, a conscious effort is made at several points in the workout to challenge the muscles with more resistance than they can comfortably handle for more than a few repetitions of the exercise. Muscles respond to the regular employment of overload challenges by steadily increasing in strength and sometimes in size as well.

In jogging or racquetball, by contrast, the degree of resistance is almost unchanged from week to week. In such activities, strength usually increases rapidly after the sport is begun but tends to plateau very quickly.

What are the benefits of weight training to those of us who have no intention of ramming a quarter ton over our heads in a weight-lifting contest or flexing "pecs" that look like living falsies in a Mr. Universe contest? There are lots of benefits, it turns out. Benefits that can help women and men—old, young and in between.

Don't expect weight training to transform an ectomorph (someone with a tall, thin frame) or an endomorph (someone with a large, heavy frame) into a mesomorph (a person of average build). "You won't change your body type," says Dr. Carnes, "but you will become the best, shapeliest example of the type you have."

Muscles help you lose weight.   Have you ever marveled at the amount of food that some teenagers can put away without showing any evidence of their gluttony? That phenomenon is often passed off as "fast metabolism," a mysterious (and wonderful) condition that just as mysteriously (and unwonderfully) becomes "slow metabolism" in the portly adult. Well, there may be some inevitability behind that sad change, but a lot of it can be attributed to fading muscles, not fading years.

Muscle tissue, you see, has a faster metabolism rate than fatty tissue, even when at rest. That means more calories are burned away, 24 hours a day.

What typically occurs after a period of weight training is that—assuming your body weight remains constant—your body gains a higher percentage of muscle and a lower percentage of fat. If you *lose* weight over a period of training, the difference is even more pronounced, because nearly all the weight you lose on a body-building program is fat, not muscle. In any event, the net result is that more of the calories you eat are being diverted to maintaining your greater proportion of muscle tissue, with fewer calories left over to cause mischief. That a 40-year-old can enjoy the metabolism of a 15-year-old is probably too much to hope for. But we do have every reason to expect that regular weight training can be of great help in stopping the weight-creep so many of us experience as adults.

How to Begin Powering Up

Let's take a look now at what weight training looks and feels like in actual practice, and how you can actually enjoy all those benefits we've talked about.

Until recently, most resistance training was carried out either in gyms devoted exclusively to weight training or in the weight rooms of Y's, which were usually not particularly attractive or comfortable. Today, however, innumerable clubs catering mostly to racquet sports have installed weight-training rooms, complete with elaborate equipment often costing tens of thousands of dollars, wall-to-wall carpeting, mirrored walls and piped-in music. Unfortunately, the one thing such rooms *don't* have is a full-time instructor or coach. Typically, there is someone to show you how to use each apparatus and perhaps to hand you a printed sheet or two with some instructions, but after that, you're pretty much on your own.

If you feel insecure about resistance training, you might want to investigate a specialized body-building studio, where you can get all the assistance you need, including gratuitous motivation in the form of men and women who have made pumping iron a way of life. On the other hand, you may find the presence of such devotees to be more intimidating than motivating—especially when the grunting and groaning begins. In which case, it's back to the weight room at the racquetball club or spa.

Another alternative is to buy your own equipment and work out at home. Many people do this quite successfully, and, especially for the first six months to a year of training, there is no reason why the results achieved should be any less impressive than those obtained at a regular gym. The major drawbacks are that many of us don't really have a suitable space to work out at home, and in order to buy the equipment necessary to exercise all parts of your body with reasonable convenience and safety, you may have to make an initial investment of anywhere from about $200 to $500.

Our advice is to begin your training at a multipurpose gym. If you decide after a few weeks that weight training isn't for you, you can always play racquetball or swim, so your investment won't be wasted. More important, perhaps, is that working out in a bright, clean, fully equipped gym is usually a lot more fun than clanking around in your basement. Fitness without fun is a recipe that often falls flat.

Besides, the diversity of weight-training equipment is so great today that it's beyond the scope of this book to tell you how to use each piece. That's a job for a knowledgeable instructor, or at least an experienced user. But what we *can* tell you is how to avoid cutting short your adventure in Hercules Land by making one or more common mistakes.

Be careful.   First realize that weights are much heavier than they look. Or even *sound.* The reason for the deceptive heaviness of weights—which is seldom appreciated—is that in our everyday activities, we usually handle heavy jobs with lots of body English, so that the muscular strain is spread out over a whole network of muscles and bones. In the gym, though, all the strain tends to be absorbed by a very localized muscle group and its associated ligaments and tendons. Joints, particularly, are vulnerable to such sharply focused strain. The trick is to begin with levels of resistance far below what you might imagine a person in your physical condition ought to be able to handle.

There is another reason for beginning with very light resistance. Although you may proceed through your first workout without any real feeling of strain, perhaps even surprising yourself at your level of ability, you may well find that the next day, or even two days after your workout, your muscles have become extremely sore. This delayed reaction to exercise stress may well bring your fitness program to a complete halt before it's even gotten under way.

When doing any resistance exercise that involves the legs or lower back, our advice is to be not just cautious but *super cautious.* The chance of eventually developing a severe muscle strain in the lower back is great.

Here are some more tips to keep you out of trouble, all from experienced weight lifters and body builders.

- When lifting any weight from the floor, always keep your back absolutely straight. And keep your neck in a straight line with your back. Don't look down at the weight; look at the wall in front of you. And put your feet as close to the weight as you can comfortably manage before lifting it. This basic technique is of crucial importance for preventing back strain.

- If you are using free weights—that is, barbells or dumbbells loaded with individual plates—make extra sure that the inside and outside collars holding the plates in place are securely locked. Even if a loose plate doesn't fall on your foot, the sudden shift of resistance and your efforts to compensate for it can bring on instant muscle strain.
- *Never* hold your breath while performing exercises against resistance. Many people do this instinctively, but it's dangerous, especially for older people. To get out of the bad habit, begin the new habit of audibly breathing in during the easy part of the exercise, then breathing out loudly during the more difficult part, such as when pressing weight over your head.
- Avoid performing any exercise in such a manner that it causes great stress in the shoulder and armpit area. Such strain occurs when, for instance, you are working with a weight-loaded bar that you pull down behind your neck from overhead. The most dangerous part of this exercise is when your arms are fully extended. In that position, a great part of the weight is no longer being handled by your muscles but by the connective tissue around your armpit. The strength of this connective tissue does not increase at anywhere near the speed of your muscles. Thus, after a few weeks, you may find yourself using levels of resistance that your back muscles can pull down but that your connective tissue can't bear when your arms are fully extended. It's a lot like putting yourself on a medieval torture rack, and an injury can be very painful and take a long time to heal.

To prevent an injury while still getting benefits from this type of exercise—an excellent one, by the way, for developing the muscles that give you a V-shaped back—follow these two tips. First, start light—use a comfortable amount of weight and do extra repetitions. When you feel ready, move to a heavier weight. Second, when doing this or any other exercise that you sense is pulling at your joints, never work with a level of resistance that forces you to put out maximum effort.

- While it's fun and helpful to your motivation to keep track of your progress, don't fall into the habit of trying to break your personal records at every workout. Although you may find yourself doing just this—successfully—for a few weeks, you must realize that unrelenting competition—even if only with yourself—is bound to result in injury.

* Unless you are extraordinarily fit, it's best to avoid lifting weights immediately after jogging. Your circulation will be severely taxed, and you will probably find yourself deeply fatigued after your workout.

* The final tip is not for the protection of your body but of your bank account. Beware of paying a full year's dues to any body-building club in advance, particularly if the club is new. That's especially true if the club is exclusively for weight training. Multipurpose athletic clubs seem to have a better record of longevity. Also, don't pay a year's dues before the place even opens on the promise of a big discount. The club may never open at all!

We're not trying to discourage you with all these words of precaution. The point is only this: The slower you go on a day-to-day basis, the faster progress you'll make month by month.

Trying to rush things will only bring on injuries that can make progress discouragingly slow. Resistance training is exercise designed for tortoises, not hares.

Warming Up

It's important that you approach any exercise routine with a series of warm-up exercises. By starting your activities slowly you accomplish three things. You warm the muscles by increasing circulation to the muscle tissue, preparing the body for vigorous exercise. You prevent injuries and soreness. And you improve your overall performance. Make five minutes of stretching a routine part of your program.

Toe Touch.   Stand with your feet together and your arms at your sides. Bend slowly at the waist, bending your knees a little at the same time, until you can grab your toes with your fingers. Stand up and repeat. (If you suffer from chronic back problems, you might want to skip the Toe Touch.)

Twist. Stand with your feet together, your back straight and your head up. Place your hands behind your head and twist your upper body left and then right, moving your elbows as far as you can to either side.

Sprinter. From a push-up position, bring one leg forward until it is under your chest and your foot is flat on the floor. Quickly change the position of your legs in a continuous movement.

Bend. Stand with your feet together and your back straight. Put your hands behind your head and bend as far as you can to the right and then to the left.

Quadriceps Stretch. Stand with your feet together and raise one leg to the rear until you can grab your ankle or your sneaker with your hand. Pull your foot toward your buttocks as far as possible without straining. Relax and repeat with the other leg. You can use a wall or a chair for balance if necessary.

Pumping Iron

The barbell and dumbbell exercises described here are designed to build muscle, improve muscular strength and endurance and firm the entire body. This combination of exercises works every major muscle.

Squat. Bend at the waist and grasp the bar in an overhand grip (palms down). Flexing your knees, stand up and curl the bar to your chest by raising your forearms only and keeping your elbows at waist level. Press it overhead and lower it to your shoulders. With your feet spread comfortably and your toes pointed outward for balance, squat slowly until your thighs are parallel to the floor. Return to the standing position. Try to keep your back and head straight throughout, and be sure to keep your feet flat on the floor.

Toe Raise. Lift the bar to your shoulders as in the squat exercise, keeping your back straight and your head up. Raise your heels off the floor as far as possible. Return to the starting position.

Curl. Stand with your back straight, your head up and your feet slightly spread. Grasp the bar in an underhand grip (palms up) with your arms fully extended. Then slowly curl the bar up to your chest.

Hold for a count of two and lower the bar slowly to the starting position. Be careful to lower the bar slowly rather than letting it drop from its own weight. Keep the bar under control at all times.

Upright Row.   Stand with your back straight and your head up. Hold the bar in an overhand grip with your arms fully extended. Keep your hands about six inches apart. Slowly raise the bar along the front of your body until your hands are under your chin. Lower the bar slowly to the starting position and repeat.

Bench Press.   Lie on your back on a bench or the floor with your back flat against the surface and the bar over your chest. Slowly press the bar straight up until your arms are fully extended, then lower it slowly to the starting position.

Triceps Extension.   Stand erect with the bar pressed straight overhead. Your hands should be about eight inches apart. Then lower the bar slowly behind your head by bending your elbows. Slowly raise the bar to the starting position and repeat.

Press behind the Neck.   Stand erect with the bar resting on your shoulders. Press the bar directly up over your head and lower it slowly to the starting position.

Dumbbell Press.   Stand with your feet comfortably spread and a dumbbell in each hand at shoulder level. Alternately press one dumbbell and then the other straight up, with your arm fully extended.

Dumbbell Swing.   Stand with your legs spread and hold a dumbbell directly over your head with both hands. Then swing the dumbbell in a wide arc down in front of you and between your legs as far as you can without straining. You'll have to bend your knees to do this properly. Reverse the process and swing the dumbbell back up to the starting position.

Shoulder Extension.   Lie flat on a bench or the floor with a dumbbell held in both hands behind your head. Keeping your arms straight, bring the dumbbell to a position over your chest. Return to the starting position.

Dumbbell Fly.   Lie flat on a bench or the floor with a dumbbell in each hand and your arms extended directly over your chest.

Slowly lower the dumbbells directly out to the sides until your arms are parallel with the floor. Then bring the dumbbells back to the starting position. Be sure to lower slowly to prevent strain on your arms.

Cooling Down

Cooling down after exercise is just as important as warming up before a workout. For one thing, your pulse rate has been elevated during exercise and it needs time to adjust to the lower demand. Cool-down exercises also help decrease muscle soreness and increase muscle flexibility. Begin these exercises with two to three minutes of walking.

Neck Stretch.   Stand with your back straight, your feet about shoulder-width apart and your arms hanging loosely at your sides. Move your head slowly to one side and hold for ten seconds, then move it to the other side and hold. Repeat, trying to bend a little farther each time.

Groin Stretch.   Sit on the floor with the soles of your feet together and your arms resting on your lower legs, with your elbows near your knees. Hold your feet together with your hands if necessary. Bend forward at the waist and slowly press your knees toward the floor with your elbows. Take it very easy and don't strain. Slowly move back to the starting position and repeat.

Swing.   Stand upright with your arms extended over your head and your legs spread. Begin to move your hands in an arc as you bend at the waist. Swing your hands between your legs as far as you can without bouncing. Touch the floor behind your heels if possible. Retrace the arc to the starting position.